Anesthesiology Pocket Guide

Anesthesiology Pocket Guide

Thomas N. Pajewski, Ph.D., M.D.
Assistant Professor of Anesthesiology and Neurological Surgery

Department of Anesthesiology
University of Virginia Health Sciences Center
Charlottesville, Virginia

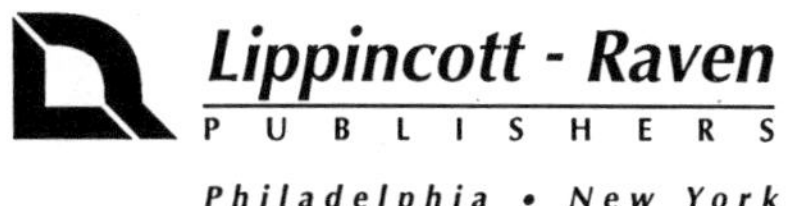

Acquisitions Editor: Craig Percy
Manufacturing Manager: Dennis Teston
Production Manager: Bernie Richey
Indexer: Mary Kidd
Printer: Victor Graphics

Printed in the United States of America 9 8 7 6 5 4 3 2 1

ISBN: 0-7817-0141-4

To my wife,
Michelle,
and
my children,
Christine and Michael

Contents

Foreword

Despite living in an age of enormous information availability, all of us experience daily the frustration of not being able to remember or to locate a pertinent bit of information that we used to know or need to know. We all have mused if only we could have taken the time earlier to collect, distill, and format for ready access information useful to us, we would not have wasted so much time later either looking for it or, not finding it, depleting a limited supply of psychic energy internally screaming about our inefficiency and coping with having to function less than fully informed. That information tidbit you so desperately require but cannot locate is now available to you in the back pocket of your scrubs. Dr. Thomas N. Pajewski has done what we all wished we were organized enough to do. He has produced a well-conceived and well-organized compendium of definitions, facts, tables, and algorithms extraordinarily useful to all of us who have responsibilities in the perioperative management of patients. When I look up a word in the dictionary, I find myself not only learning the definition of that word but of several others also. My experience using this pocket guide is very much the same. Not only do I easily find the information I seek, I also read several other pages in close proximity. Continuing medical education and sangfroid. What more could I ask. I will wear this book out. I think you will too.

Raymond C. Roy, Ph.D., M.D.
Distinguished Professor & Chair
Department of Anesthesiology
University of Virginia Health Sciences Center
Charlottesville, Virginia

Preface

This book was developed from the realization that frequently one is faced with a situation where a specific fact or drug dose is needed, but is not readily available. While we are not always able to easily reference our favorite anesthesiology textbooks or relevant journals when working in the OR or in an intensive care unit, many of us have developed notebooks or notecards to keep track of particularly useful tables and figures. This book grew out of such an exercise. There are numerous handbooks available for those of us interested in the practice of anesthesiology. Many of them contain an extensive amount of information including lengthy description of medical situations or procedures, however, much of the time that piece of information so desperately needed cannot be quickly extracted and put to use. This book is an example of an organized collection of information relevant to the practice of anesthesiology. It is hoped that it will find use as a valuable companion for not only anesthesiology residents, medical students and nurse anesthetists, but also the more experienced practitioner who likes to have ready access to the information contained herein.

Acknowledgments

I would like to acknowledge the assistance of my many colleagues who helped in offering suggestions and in reviewing this book. In particular, I would like to thank Todd G. Hermann, M.D., Jennifer E. O'Flaherty, M.D., MPH, and especially B. Todd Sitzman, M.D., MPH for their invaluable and much appreciated effort in reviewing the material in this book and for offering insightful criticism.

Preoperative Considerations

Preoperative Assessment

American Society of Anesthesiologists Physical Status Classification

Class	Description
1	A normal healthy patient
2	A patient with mild systemic disease (e.g., anemia, controlled essential hypertension, well-controlled mild diabetes)
3	A patient with severe systemic disease that limits activity (e.g., stable angina pectoris, prior myocardial infarction, severely limiting organic heart disease, moderate pulmonary insufficiency, severe diabetes)
4	A patient with severe systemic disease that is a constant threat to life (e.g., unstable angina pectoris, organic heart disease with evidence of failure, advanced degrees of endocrine, hepatic, pulmonary or renal insufficiency)
5	A moribund patient who is not expected to survive longer than 24 hours without the operation (e.g., massive cerebral trauma with rapidly increasing intracranial pressure, ruptured abdominal aortic aneurysm with severe hemodynamic instability, massive pulmonary embolism)
6	A declared brain-dead patient whose organs are being removed for donor purposes
E	Placed as a suffix to the physical status designation for emergency patients (for example, 2E)

Perioperative Mortality Rates

Class	Mortality Rate (per 10,000 patients)
1	6 - 8
2	27 - 40
3	180 - 430
4	780 - 2300
5	940 - 5100

(based on ASA Physical Status Classification)

Suggested Preoperative Laboratory Tests

Test	**Patient Population**
Electrocardiogram	Patients over 40 years old
Blood Work	
Hemoglobin or hematocrit	Menstruating women
	Patients over 60 years old
	Patients likely to experience significant blood loss and may require blood transfusion
Creatinine (or blood urea nitrogen)	Patients over 60 years old
Serum glucose	Patients over 60 years old
Chest radiograph	Patients over 60 years old

These guidelines assume that the patient is apparently healthy and asymptomatic.

Other tests should be guided the history and physical examination of the patient (e.g., serum potassium in a patient taking a diuretic for blood pressure control).

These guidelines focus on a patient's age as the primary determinant for which tests are likely to yield clinically significant information.

An alternative approach is presented in the following table.

Recommended Preoperative Screening Tests for Selected Medical Situations

Medical Condition	Preoperative Screening Tests
Cardiovascular disease	BUN, creatinine, CXR, ECG, Hgb
Pulmonary disease	CXR, ECG, possible ABG
Renal disease	Electrolytes, BUN, creatinine, Hgb, platelet count
Hepatic disease	PT, PTT, SGOT, alkaline phosphatase, platelet count
Diabetes	Electrolytes, platelet count, glucose, ECG, BUN, creatinine
Hypertension	ECG, BUN, creatinine, electrolytes with diuretic usage
Seizure disorder	Serum anti-convulsant level
Possible pregnancy	β-HCG
Steroid usage	Blood glucose, platelet count

Use of Prior Test Results

Chest x-ray	A chest X-ray showing normal results that was performed within one year of surgery can be used if there has been no intervening clinical event.
ECG	An ECG showing normal results that was performed within six months of surgery can be used if there has been no intervening clinical event.
Blood Tests	Tests performed within six weeks of surgery that show normal results can be used if there has been no intervening clinical event.

Reprinted with permission from reference 1.

New York Heart Association's Functional Classification of Patients with Cardiac Disease

Class	Description
Class I:	No limitation of physical activity. Ordinary physical activity does not cause symptoms such as undue fatigue, palpitations, dyspnea or angina.
Class II:	Slight limitation of physical activity. Comfortable at rest but ordinary physical activity results in symptoms.
Class III:	Marked limitation of physical activity. Comfortable at rest but less than ordinary physical activity results in symptoms.
Class IV:	Inability to carry on any physical activity without discomfort. Symptoms of cardiac insufficiency or of anginal syndrome may be present even at rest. If any physical activity is undertaken, discomfort is increased.

Grading of Heart Murmurs

Grade	Description
I/VI	Heard only after special maneuvers and "tuning in"
II/VI	Faint, but readily heard
III/VI	Loud, but without a thrill
IV/VI	Associated with a thrill, but stethoscope must be fully on chest to be heard
V/VI	Heard with stethoscope partly off the chest, palpable thrill
VI/VI	Heard with stethoscope entirely off the chest, palpable thrill

Grading of Pulses

Grade	Description
0	Pulse absent
1+	Diminished amplitude, weak
2+	Normal
3+	Hyperkinetic
4+	Bounding, excessive

Grading of Edema

Grade	Description
0	Absent, no pit
1+	Normal contour, slight pit
2+	Fairly normal contour, persistent pit
3+	Abnormal contour, deep pitting
4+	Skin leaks fluid from any breaks

Grading of Reflex Intensity

Grade 0	0	Absent
Grade 1	+	Diminished but present
Grade 2	++	Normal
Grade 3	+++	Brisker than average but probably normal
Grade 4	++++	Hyperactive often with clonus

Locating The Myocardial Infarct

Area of Infarct	Affected ECG Leads
Anterior	I, aVL, V_3, V_4
Inferior	II, III, aVF
Lateral	I, aVL, V_5, V_6
Posterior	Reciprocal changes in V_1, V_2
Anterolateral	V_{1-6}
Anteroseptal	V_{1-4}
Inferolateral	Inferior + V_5, V_6
Right Ventricle	V_{4R}-V_{6R}

Reproduced with permission from reference 2.

ECG Changes Associated With Electrolyte Abnormalities

Electrolyte Change	ECG Response
Hypokalemia	ST-segment depression T wave flattening and inversion Tall U wave
Hyperkalemia	Tall T wave P-R interval prolongation ST-segment depression QRS widening Ventricular fibrillation
Hypocalcemia	Prolonged QT interval
Hypercalcemia	Short QT interval ST segment may disappear

Reproduced with permission from reference 2.

Different Lead Combinations for Ischemia Detection

Combination	Lead(s)	% Sensitivity
One lead	II	33
	V_4	61
	V_5	75
Two leads	II / V_5	80
	II / V_4	82
	V_4 / V_5	90
Three leads	V_3 / V_4 / V_5	94
	II / V_4 / V_5	96
Four leads	II / V_3 - V_5	100

Reproduced with permission from reference 3.

Computation of the Cardiac Risk Index (Goldman Criteria)

Criteria*	"Points"
1. History:	
(a) Age >70 yr	5
(b) MI in previous 6 months	10
2. Physical examination:	
(a) S_3 gallop or JVD	11
(b) Important VAS	3
3. Electrocardiogram:	
(a) Rhythm other than sinus or PAC's on last preoperative ECG	7
(b) >5 PVC's/min documented at any time before operation	7
4. General status: PO_2 <60 or PCO_2 >50 mm Hg, K+ <3.0 or HCO_3 <20 mEq/liter, BUN >50 or Cr >3.0 mg/dl, abnormal SGOT, signs of chronic liver disease or patient bed ridden from noncardiac causes	3
5. Operation:	
(a) Intraperitoneal, intrathoracic or aortic operation	3
(b) Emergency operation	4
Total possible	53 points

*MI denotes myocardial infarction, JVD jugular-vein distention, VAS valvular aortic stenosis, PAC's premature atrial contractions, ECG electrocardiogram, PVC's premature ventricular contractions, PO_2 partial pressure of oxygen, PCO_2 partial pressure of carbon dioxide, K+ potassium, HCO_3 bicarbonate, BUN blood urea nitrogen, Cr creatinine & SGOT serum glutamic oxalacetic transaminase.

Class	Point Total	Risk Assessment
I	0 - 5	Routine preoperative medical consultation from a cardiac risk standpoint is not indicated.
II	6 - 12	Routine preoperative medical consultation from a cardiac risk standpoint probably not indicated.
III	13 - 25	These patients probably have sufficient cardiac risk to warrant routine preoperative medical consultation from a cardiac risk standpoint.
IV	≥ 26	Only truly life-saving procedures should be performed on these patients.

Reproduced with permission from reference 4.

Note: There are other indexes used to evaluate cardiac risk.
Detsky AS et al. J Gen Intern Med 1986;1:211-9
Larsen SF et al. Eur Heart J 1987;8:179-85

Clinical Predictors of Increased Perioperative Cardiovascular Risk (Myocardial Infarction, Congestive Heart Failure, Death)

Major

Unstable coronary syndromes

- Recent myocardial infarction* with evidence of important ischemic risk by clinical symptoms or noninvasive study
- Unstable or severe† angina (Canadian Class III or IV)

Decompensated congestive heart failure

Significant arrhythmias

- High-grade atrioventricular block
- Symptomatic ventricular arrhythmias in the presence of underlying heart disease
- Supraventricular arrhythmias with uncontrolled ventricular rate

Severe valvular disease

Intermediate

Mild angina pectoris (Canadian Class I or II)

Prior myocardial infarction by history or pathological Q waves

Compensated or prior congestive heart failure

Diabetes mellitus

Minor

Advanced age

Abnormal ECG (left ventricular hypertrophy, left bundle branch block, ST-T abnormalities)

Rhythm other than sinus (e.g., atrial fibrillation)

Low functional capacity (e.g., inability to climb one flight of stairs with a bag of groceries)

History of stroke

Uncontrolled systemic hypertension

ECG indicates electrocardiogram.

*The American College of Cardiology National Database Library defines recent MI as greater than 7 days but less than or equal to 1 month (30 days).

†May include "stable" angina in patients who are unusually sedentary.

Reproduced with permission from reference 5.

Cardiac Risk* Stratification for Noncardiac Surgical Procedures

High (Reported cardiac risk often >5%)

- Emergent major operations, particularly in the elderly
- Aortic and other major vascular
- Peripheral vascular
- Anticipated prolonged surgical procedures associated with large fluid shifts and/or blood loss

Intermediate (Reported cardiac risk generally <5%)

- Carotid endarterectomy
- Head and neck
- Intraperitoneal and intrathoracic
- Orthopedic
- Prostate

Low† (Reported cardiac risk generally <1 %)

- Endoscopic procedures
- Superficial procedure
- Cataract
- Breast

*Combined incidence of cardiac death and nonfatal myocardial infarction.
†Do not generally require further preoperative cardiac testing.

Reproduced with permission from reference 5.

Prognostic Gradient of Ischemic Responses During an ECG-Monitored Exercise Test

Patients with suspected or proven CAD

High Risk

Ischemia induced by low-level exercise† (<4 METs or heart rate <100 bpm or <70% age predicted) manifested by one or more of the following:

- Horizontal or downsloping ST depression >0.1 mV
- ST-segment elevation >0.1 mV in noninfarct lead
- Five or more abnormal leads
- Persistent ischemic response >3 min after exertion
- Typical angina

Intermediate Risk

Ischemia induced by moderate-level exercise (4 - 6 METs or heart rate 100 - 130 bpm [70 - 85% age predicted] manifested by one or more of the following:

- Horizontal or downsloping ST depression >0.1 mV
- Typical angina
- Persistent ischemic response >1-3 min after exertion
- Three to four abnormal leads

Low Risk

No ischemia or ischemia induced at high-level exercise. (>7 METs or heart rate >130 bpm [>85% age predicted) manifested by:

- Horizontal or downsloping ST depression >0.1 mV
- Typical angina
- One to two abnormal leads

Inadequate Test

Inability to reach adequate target workload or heart rate response for age without an ischemic response. For patients undergoing noncardiac surgery, ability to exercise to at least the intermediate-risk level without ischemia should be considered at low risk for perioperative ischemic events.

ECG indicates electrocardiographically; MET, metabolic equivalent; bpm, beats per minute.

†Workload and heart rate estimates for risk severity require adjustment for patient age. Maximum target heart rates for 40- and 80-year-old subjects on no cardioactive medication are 180 and 140 beats per minute respectively.

Reproduced with permission from reference 5.

Estimated Energy Requirements for Various Activities

1 MET	Can you take care of yourself?
↓	Eat, dress, or use the toilet?
↓	Walk indoors around the house?
↓ ↓	Walk a block or two on level ground? at 2 - 3 mph or 3.2 - 4.8 km/h?
↓ ↓	Do light work around the house like dusting or washing dishes?
4 METS	Climb a flight of stairs or walk up a hill?
↓	Walk on level ground at 4 mph or 6.4 km/hr?
↓	Run a short distance?
↓ ↓	Do heavy work around the house like scrubbing floors or lifting or moving heavy furniture?
↓ ↓ ↓	Particpate in moderate recreational activities like golf, bowling, dancing, doubles tennis, or throwing a baseball or football?
≥10 METs	Participate in strenuous sports like swimming singles tennis, football, basketball, or skiing?

MET indicates metabolic equivalent.

Reproduced with permission from reference 5.

Indications for Coronary Angiography* in Perioperative Evaluation Before (or After) Noncardiac Surgery

Class I†: Patients with suspected or proven CAD:

- High-risk results during noninvasive testing
- Angina pectoris unresponsive to adequate medical therapy
- Most patients with unstable angina pectoris
- Nondiagnostic or equivocal noninvasive test in a high-risk patient undergoing a high-risk noncardiac surgical procedure

Class II†:

- Intermediate-risk results during noninvasive testing
- Nondiagnostic or equivocal noninvasive test in a lower-risk patient undergoing a high-risk noncardiac surgical procedure
- Urgent noncardiac surgery in a patient convalescing from acute MI
- Perioperative MI

Class III†:

- Low-risk noncardiac surgery in a patient with known CAD and low-risk results on noninvasive testing
- Screening for CAD without appropriate noninvasive testing
- Asymptomatic after coronary revascularization, with excellent exercise capacity (≥7 METs)
- Mild stable angina in patients with good LV function, low-risk noninvasive test results
- Patient is not a candidate for coronary revascularization because of concomitant medical illness
- Prior technically adequate normal coronary angiogram within 5 years
- Severe LV dysfunction (eg, ejection fraction <20%) and patient not considered candidate for revascularization procedure
- Patient unwilling to consider coronary revascularization procedure

*If results will affect management.

†Class I: Conditions for which there is evidence for and/or general agreement that a procedure be performed or a treatment is of benefit. Class II: Conditions for which there is a divergence of evidence and/or opinion about the treatment. Class III: Conditions for which there is evidence and/or general agreement that the procedure is not necessary.

CAD indicates coronary artery disease; MI, myocardial infarction; MET, metabolic equivalent; LV, left ventricular.

Reprinted with permission from reference 5.

Recommendations for Perioperative Cardiac Evaluation and Management for Major Noncardiac Surgery

Characteristics of Patients*	Preoperative Diagnostic Testing	Special Perioperative Treatment
No known coronary artery disease Good cardiac functional status Class I-II on the cardiac risk index or low risk on other validated indexes (regardless of risk factors for coronary artery disease or type of surgery)	None except routine 12-lead electrocardiography and chest radiography	None†
Known stable coronary artery disease with good functional status (class I or early class II)	None except routine 12-lead electrocardiography and chest radiography	Conservative treatment: Continue cardiac medications Postoperative electrocardiogram on day I and to rule out myocardial infarction after any suspicious perioperative events, and again before hospital discharge
Known coronary artery disease, functional status unclear	Noninvasive testing Exercise stress testing if patient can exercise Other tests (dipyridamole-thallium scintigraphy, stress echocardiography, or ambulatory monitoring for ischemia) if patient cannot exercise	If test is negative: conservative treatment (see above) If test is positive: aggressive medical treatment or angiography Intensify preoperative medications for coronary artery disease, identify and address cardiac and noncardiac risk factors, and consider repeating noninvasive testing if major changes have been made; if tests are negative, use

		conservative treatment; if still positive, proceed to: More intensive perioperative monitoring and perioperative medications to control blood pressure and pulse or Coronary angiography and revascularization as indicated
Known coronary artery disease, poor cardiac functional status	None	Aggressive medical treatment or angiography (see above)
Poor noncardiac functional status, no coronary artery disease, or status unclear		
No or few risk factors‡	None	None
Multiple risk factors‡	Noninvasive testing (see above)	If test is negative: conservative treatment (see above) If test is positive: aggressive medical treatment or angiography (see above)
Coronary artery disease and either class III or IV on the cardiac risk index or high risk on other validated indexes	None	Aggressive medical treatment or angiography (see above)

See following page for further explanations.

Recommendations for Perioperative Cardiac Evaluation and Management for Major Noncardiac Surgery (continued)

*Coronary artery disease is defined by a clinical diagnosis of angina, a prior myocardial infarction, or a positive coronary angiogram Functional class I or II indicates that the patient can walk up a flight of stairs carrying a bag of groceries or perform an equivalent activity without cardiac symptoms.

†Cardiac medications should generally be continued before surgery and resumed as soon as possible thereafter. Intravenous formulations or substitutes should be used in patients who require medications that cannot be given orally in the perioperative period. Intraoperative and postoperative techniques should be chosen to modulate sympathetic responses. Some procedures may require specialized monitoring independent of a patient s cardiac status. Pulmonary-artery catheterization is often recommended for monitoring patients with very advanced heart failure, aortic stenosis, or a recent myocardial infarction (occurring less than four to six weeks earlier), and for those undergoing abdominal or thoracic aortic surgery

‡Risk factors include an age over 70, diabetes mellitus, congestive heart failure, important atrial or ventricular arrhythmias, known vascular disease, and the need for aortic, abdominal, or thoracic surgery.

Reprinted with permission from reference 6.

Indications for Implantation of Permanent Pacemakers for Bradycardia in Adults

Acquired AV Heart Block

Class I: Permanent or intermittent third-degree block with symptomatic bradycardia or congestive heart failure. Ectopic rhythms or medical conditions requiring bradycardic drugs. Asystole ≥ 3.0 second or escape rate < 40 beats/min without symptoms. Post AV junctional ablation, or myotonic dystrophy. Type I or II, second-degree AV block with symptomatic bradycardia. Atrial flutter-fibrillation or SVT with advanced second or third-degree AV block and symptomatic bradycardia not due to drugs.

Class II: Asymptomatic third-degree AV block with rates > 40 beats/min. Asymptomatic type II, second-degree AV block. Asymptomatic type I, second-degree AV block at or below the common (His) bundle.

Class III: Asymptomatic first-degree AV block. Type I, second-degree AV block at the AV node.

AV Block After Myocardial Infarction

Class I: Persistent advanced second- or third-degree AV block with block in the His-Purkinje system. Patients with transient advanced second-degree AV block and bundle branch block.

Class II: Patients with persistent advanced second-degree AV block at the AV node.

Class III: Transient AV conduction disturbances without intraventricular conduction defects. Transient AV block with isolated left anterior hemiblock, or the latter without AV block. Persistent first-degree AV block in the presence of bundle branch block not demonstrated previously.

Chronic Bifascicular and Trifascicular Block

Class I: Bifascicular or trifascicular block with intermittent third-degree AV block and symptomatic bradycardia or intermittent type II, second-degree AV block with symptoms attributable to heart block.

Class II: Bifascicular or trifascicular block with syncope that cannot be attributed to third-degree AV block or other causes. Prolonged HV interval (≥ 100 msec) or pacing-induced infra-His block.

Class III: Fascicular block (+ first-degree AV block) without type II second degree AV block or symptoms.

Sinus Node Dysfunction

Class I: SND with documented symptomatic bradycardia, including that consequent to chronic, essential drug therapy for which there are not acceptable alternatives.

Class II: Spontaneous or drug-induced SND with heart rates < 40 beats/min when there is no clear association between symptoms of bradycardia and the occurrence of bradycardia.

Hypersensitive Carotid Sinus and Neurovascular Syndromes

Class I: Recurrent syncope associated with clear, spontaneous events provoked by carotid sinus stimulation. Minimal carotid sinus pressure induces asystole > 3 seconds in the absence of drugs that depress sinus or AV node function.

Class II: Recurrent syncope without clear, provocative events, and with a hypersensitive cardioinhibitory response. Syncope with associated bradycardia reproduced by provocative maneuvers (e.g., head-up tilt + isoproterenol), and in which temporary pacing and a second provocative test establish the likely benefits of permanent pacing.

Class III: Hyperactive cardioinhibitory response with or without vague symptoms such as dizziness or lightheadedness or both. Recurrent syncope, dizziness, lightheadedness in the absence of a cardioinhibitory response.

Definitions

Class I Conditions for which there is general agreement that permanent pacemakers or antitachycardia devices should be implanted.

Class II Conditions for which permanent pacemakers or antitachycardia devices are frequently used, but about which there is divergence of opinion with respect to the necessity of their insertion.

Class III Conditions for which there is general agreement that pacemakers or antitachycardia devices are unnecessary.

AV heart block is defined as follows:

1. First-degree AV block is PR-interval prolongation without dropped beats
2. Type I (Wenckebach) second-degree AV block is increasing PR-interval prolongation with dropped beats
3. Type II (Mobitz) second-degree AV block is intermittent dropped beats without PR-interval prolongation.
4. Advanced second-degree AV block is two or more successive dropped beats with some conducted beats.
5. Third-degree or complete AV block is no conducted beats from the atrium.

Intraventricular heart block is defined as a conduction block within or anywhere below the common (His) bundle.

Fascicular heart block is defined as a conduction block occurring the right bundle branch or the two major divisions of the left bundle branch.

HV interval is defined as the onset of His deflection to beginning of ventricular electrogram in His bundle electrogram.

Adapted from reference 7.

Indications for Pacing in Children with Bradycardia or AV Heart Block

Class I Indications

1. Second- or third-degree AV heart block, or SND, with symptomatic bradycardia.
2. Advanced second- or third-degree AV block with moderate exercise intolerance.
3. Congenital AV block and wide SIRS escape rhythm or intraventricular block.
4. Advanced second- or third-degree AV block 10 to 14 days following cardiac surgery.

Class II Indications

1. Brady-tachy syndrome if digitalis or phenytoin does not control arrhythmias.
2. Second- or third-degree AV block within common bundle in asymptomatic patient.
3. Transient surgical second- or third-degree AV block that reverts to bifascicular block.
4. Asymptomatic second- or third-degree AV block and ventricular rate < 45 beats/min (awake).
5. Complete AV block with average ventricular rate < 50 beats/min (awake).
6. Asymptomatic neonate, congenital third-degree AV block and bradycardia.*
7. Complex ventricular arrhythmias with second- or third-degree AV block or sinus bradycardia.
8. Congenital long-QT syndrome for prophylaxis of torsades de pointes VT.

Class III Indications

1. Asymptomatic, postoperative bifascicular block with or without first degree AV block.
2. Transient surgical AV block that returns to normal conduction in < 1 week.
3. Asymptomatic congenital heart block without profound bradycardia.*

Definitions

Class I — Conditions for which there is general agreement that permanent pacemakers or antitachycardia devices should be implanted.

Class II — Conditions for which permanent pacemakers or antitachycardia devices are frequently used, but about which there is divergence of opinion with respect to the necessity of their insertion.

Class III — Conditions for which there is general agreement that pacemakers or antitachycardia devices are unnecessary.

*Bradycardia in relation to normal values for children with congenital heart block and same age. Adapted from reference 7.

Indications for Permanent Antitachyarrhythmia Pacing Devices

Devices that Automatically Detect and Pace to Terminate Tachycardias

Class 1: Symptomatic recurrent SVT when drugs fail to control the arrhythmia or produce intolerable side effects, and catheter or surgical ablation failed or refused. Symptomatic recurrent VT with ICD back-up if recurrent VT is not prevented by drugs and no other therapy is available.

Class II: Pacing for recurrent SVT in place of drugs or other treatment.

Class III: Tachycardias that accelerate/convert to fibrillation with pacing.

External, Manually Activated Devices to Terminate Tachycardia

Class I: Recurrent symptomatic VT uncontrolled by drugs when surgery, catheter ablation or ICD/automatic device implantation is not indicated.

Class III: Recurrent SVT or VT that produces syncope.

Overdrive or Atrial Synchronous Pacemakers to Prevent Tachycardia

Class I: AV or AV node reentrant SVT not responsive to medical therapy.

Class II: Sustained VT if other therapies are ineffective or inapplicable and efficacy of pacing is thoroughly documented. Long-QT syndrome.

Class III: Frequent or complex ventricular ectopy without sustained VT associated with coronary artery disease, cardiomyopathy, mitral valve prolapse, or abnormal heart in the absence of the long-QT syndrome. Long-QT syndrome due to remediable causes.

Definitions

Class I	Conditions for which there is general agreement that permanent pacemakers or antitachycardia devices should be implanted.
Class II	Conditions for which permanent pacemakers or antitachycardia devices are frequently used, but about which there is divergence of opinion with respect to the necessity of their insertion.
Class III	Conditions for which there is general agreement that pacemakers or antitachycardia devices are unnecessary.

Adapted from reference 7.

Prevention of Wound Infection and Sepsis in Surgical Patients

Name of Operation	Likely Pathogen	Recommended Drugs	Adult Dosage Before Surgery (1)
CLEAN			
Cardiac			
Prosthetic valve, coronary artery bypass, other open heart surgery, pacemaker implant	*Staphylococcus epidermidis*, *S. aureus*, Corynebacterium, enteric gram-negative bacilli	cefazolin or cefuroxime OR vancomycin **(3)**	1-2 grams IV(**2**) 1 gram IV
Vascular			
Arterial surgery involving the abdominal aorta, a prosthesis, or a groin incision	*S. aureus*, *S. epidermidis*, enteric gram-negative bacilli	cefazolin OR vancomycin **(3)**	1-2 grams IV 1 gram IV
Lower extremity amputation for ischemia	*S. aureus*, *S. epidermidis*, enteric gram-negative bacilli, clostridia	cefazolin OR vancomycin **(3)**	1 gram IV 1 gram IV
Neurosurgery			
Craniotomy	*S. aureus*, *S. epidermidis*	cefazolin OR vancomycin **(3)**	1 gram IV 1 gram IV
Orthopedic			
Total joint replacement, internal fixation of fractures	*S. aureus*, *S. epidermidis*	cefazolin OR vancomycin **(3)**	1-2 gram IV 1 gram IV
Ophthalmic	*S. aureus*, *S. epidermidis*, streptococci, enteric gram-negative bacilli, *Pseudomonas*	gentamicin OR tobramycin OR neomycin-gramicidin-polymyxin B cefazolin	multiple drops topically over 2 to 24 hours 100 mg subconjunctivally at the end of procedure

Name of Operation	Likely Pathogen	Recommended Drugs	Adult Dosage Before Surgery (1)
CLEAN-CONTAMINATED			
Head and neck			
Entering oral cavity oropharynx	*S. aureus*, streptococci, oral anaerobes	cefazolin OR clindamycin	1-2 grams IV 600-900 mg IV
Abdominal			
Gastroduodenal	Enteric gram-negative bacilli, gram positive cocci	High risk, gastric bypass, or percutaneous endoscopic gastrostomy only: cefazolin	1 gram IV
Biliary tract	Enteric gram-negative bacilli, enterococci, clostridia	High risk only: cefazolin	1 gram IV
Colorectal	Enteric gram-negative bacilli, anaerobes	Oral: neomycin + erythromycin base **(4)** Parenteral: cefoxitin OR cefotetan	 1 gram IV
Appendectomy	Enteric gram-negative bacilli, anaerobes	cefoxitin OR cefotetan	1 gram IV
Gynecologic			
Vaginal or abdominal hysterectomy	Enteric gram-negatives, anaerobes, Group B. strep, enterococci	cefazolin	1 gram IV
Cesarean section	same as hysterectomy	High risk only: cefazolin	1 gram IV after cord clamping
Abortion	same as for hysterectomy	First trimester high risk **(5)** aqueous penicillin G OR doxycycline Second trimester: cefazolin	 1 million units IV 300 mg PO **(6)** 1 gram IV

Prevention of Wound Infection and Sepsis in Surgical Patients (continued)

Name of Operation	Likely Pathogen	Recommended Drugs	Adult Dosage Before Surgery (1)
DIRTY SURGERY			
Ruptured viscus **(7)**	Enteric gram-negative bacilli, anaerobes, enterococci	cefoxitin	2 grams IV q 6 h
		OR cefotetan	1-2 grams IV q 12 h
		either ± gentamicin	1.5 mg/kg IV q 8 h
		OR clindamycin	600 mg IV q 6 h
		+ gentamicin	1.5 mg/kg IV q 8 h
Traumatic wound **(7,8)**	*S. aureus*, Group A strep, clostridia	cefazolin	1-2 grams IV q 8 h

1. Parenteral prophylactic antimicrobials can be given as a single dose intravenously just before the operation. Cefazolin can also be given intramuscularly. For prolonged operations, additional intraoperative doses should be given q 4-8 h for the duration of the procedure.
2. Some consultants recommend an additional dose when patients are removed from bypass during open-heart surgery.
3. For hospitals in which methicillin-resistant *S. aureus* and *S. epidermidis* frequently cause wound infection, or for patients allergic to penicillins or cephalosporins. Rapid IV administration may cause hypotension, which could be especially dangerous during induction of anesthesia. Even if the drug is given over 60 minutes, hypotension may occur; treatment with diphenhydramine (Benadryl and others) and further slowing of the infusion rate may be helpful (DG Maki et al, J Thorac Cardiovasc Surg, 104:1423, 1992). For procedures in which enteric gram-negative bacilli are likely pathogens, such as vascular surgery involving a groin incision, cefazolin should be included in the prophylaxis regimen.
4. After appropriate diet and catharsis, one gram of each at 1 PM, 2 PM, and 11 PM the day before an 8 AM operation.
5. Patients with previous pelvic inflammatory disease, previous gonorrhea, or multiple sex partners.
6. Divided into 100 mg one hour before the abortion and 200 mg one half hour after.
7. For "dirty" surgery, therapy should usually be continued for five to 10 days.
8. For bite wounds, in which likely pathogens may also include oral anaerobes, *Eikenella corrodens* (human), and *Pasteurella* multocide (dog and cat), some Medical Letter consultants recommend use of amoxicillin-clavulanic acid (*Augmentin*) or ampicillin-sulbactam (*Unasyn*).

Prevention of Bacterial Endocarditis; Recommendations by the American Heart Association Recommendations on Endocarditis Prophylaxis - Cardiac Conditions*

Endocarditis Prophylaxis Recommended	Endocarditis Prophylaxis Not Recommended
Prosthetic cardiac valves, including bioprosthetic and homograft valves	Isolated secundum atrial septal defect
Previous bacterial endocarditis, even in the absence of heart disease	Cardiac pacemakers and implanted defibrillators
Most congenital cardiac malformations	Previous coronary artery bypass graft surgery
Mitral valve prolapse with valvular regurgitation	Mitral valve prolapse without valvular regurgitation**
Hypertrophic cardiomyopathy	Physiologic, functional, or innocent heart murmur
Rheumatic and other acquired valvular dysfunction, even after valvular surgery	Previous Kawasaki disease without valvular dysfunction
	Previous rheumatic fever without valvular dysfunction
	Surgical repair with residual beyond 6 month of secundum atrial septal defect, ventricular septal defect, or patent ductus arteriosus

* This table lists selected conditions but is not meant to be all-inclusive.

** Individuals who have a mitral valve prolapse associated with thickening and/or redundancy of the valve leaflets may be at increased for bacterial endocarditis, particularly men who are 45 years or older.

Reproduced with permission from reference 9.

Recommendations on Endocarditis Prophylaxis - Dental or Surgical Procedures*

Endocarditis Prophylaxis Recommended	Endocarditis Prophylaxis Not Recommended**
Dental procedures known to induce gingival or mucosal bleeding, including professional cleaning	Dental procedures not likely to induce gingival or mucosal bleeding, such as simple adjustment of orthodontic appliances or fillings above the gum line
Tonsillectomy and/or adenoidectomy	Injection of local intraoral anesthetic (except intraligamentary injections)
Surgical operations that involve intestinal or respiratory mucosa	Shedding of primary teeth
Bronchoscopy with a rigid bronchoscope	Tympanostomy tube insertion
Sclerotherapy of esophageal varices	Endotracheal intubation
Esophageal dilation	Bronchoscopy with a flexible bronchoscope, with or without biopsy
Gallbladder surgery	Cardiac catheterization
Cystoscopy	Endoscopy with or without gastrointestinal biopsy
Urethral dilation	Cesarean section
Urethral catheterization if urinary tract infection is present***	In the absence of infection for urethral catheterization, dilatation and curettage, uncomplicated vaginal delivery, therapeutic abortion, sterilization procedures, or insertion or removal of intrauterine devices
Urinary tract surgery if urinary tract infection is present***	
Prostatic surgery	
Incision and drainage of infected tissue***	
Vaginal hysterectomy	
Vaginal delivery in the presence of infection***	

* This table lists selected conditions but is not meant to be all-inclusive.

** In patients who have prosthetic heart valves, a previous history of endocarditis, or surgically constructed systemic-pulmonary shunts or conduits, physicians may choose to administer prophylactic antibiotics even for low-risk procedures that involve the lower respiratory, genitourinary, or gastrointestinal tracts.

*** In addition to the prophylactic regimen for genitourinary procedures, antibiotic therapy should be directed against the most likely bacterial pathogen.

Recommended Standard Prophylactic Regimen for Dental, Oral, or Upper Respiratory Tract Procedures in Patients Who Are at Risk*

Drug	Dosing Regimen**
Standard Regimen	
Amoxicillin	3.0 gm orally 1 h before procedure, then 1.5 gm 6 h after initial dose
Amoxicillin/Penicillin-Allergic Patients	
Erythromycin	Erythromycin ethylsuccinate, 800 mg, or erythromycin stearate 1.0 gm orally 2 h before procedure, then half the dose 6 h after initial dose
or	
Clindamycin	300 mg orally 1 h before procedure and 150 mg 6 h after initial dose

* Includes those with prosthetic heart valves and other high-risk patients.

** Initial pediatric doses are as follows: amoxicillin, 50 mg/kg; erythromycin ethylsuccinate or erythromycin stearate, 20 mg/kg; and clindamycin, 10 mg/kg. Follow-up doses should be one-half the initial dose. Total pediatric dose should not exceed total adult dose. The following weight range may also be used for the initial pediatric dose of amoxicillin: <15 kg, 750 mg; 15 to 30 kg, 1500 mg; and >30 kg, 3000 mg (full adult dose).

Reproduced with permission from reference 9.

Alternate Prophylactic Regimens for Dental, Oral, or Upper Respiratory Tract Procedures in Patients Who Are at Risk

Drug	Dosing Regimen*
Patients Unable to Take Oral Medications	
Ampicillin	Intravenous or intramuscular administration of ampicillin 2.0 gm, 30 min before procedure, then intravenous or intramuscular administration of ampicillin, 1.0 gm, or oral administration of amoxicillin, 1.5 gm, 6 h after initial dose
Ampicillin/Amoxicillin/Penicillin-Allergic Patients Unable to Take Oral Medications	
Clindamycin	Intravenous administration of 300 mg 30 min before procedure and an intravenous or oral administration of 150 mg 6 h after initial dose
Patients Considered High Risk and Not Candidates for Standard Regimen	
Ampicillin, gentamycin, and amoxicillin	Intravenous or intramuscular administration of ampicillin 2.0 gm, plus gentamicin, 1.5 mg/kg (not to exceed 80 mg), 30 min before procedure; followed by amoxicillin, 1.5 gm, orally 8 h after initial dose; alternatively, the parenteral regimen may be repeated 8 h after initial dose
Ampicillin/Amoxicillin/Penicillin-Allergic Patients Considered High Risk	
Vancomycin	Intravenous administration of 1.0 gm over 1 h, starting 1 h before procedure; no repeat dose necessary

* Initial pediatric doses are as follows: ampicillin, 50 mg/kg; clindamycin, 10 mg/kg; gentamycin, 2.0 mg/kg; and vancomycin 20 mg/kg. Follow-up doses should be one half of the initial dose. Total pediatric dose should not exceed total adult dose. No initial dose is recommended in this table for amoxicillin (25 mg/kg is the follow-up dose).

Regimens for Genitourinary/Gastrointestinal Procedures

Drug	Dosage Regimen*
Standard Regimen	
Ampicillin, gentamycin, and amoxicillin	Intravenous or intramuscular administration of ampicillin 2.0 gm, plus gentamicin, 1.5 mg/kg (not to exceed 80 mg), 30 min before procedure; followed by amoxicillin, 1.5 gm, orally 8 h after initial dose; alternatively, the parenteral regimen may be repeated 8 h after initial dose
Ampicillin/Amoxicillin/Penicillin-Allergic Patients Regimen	
Vancomycin and gentamycin	Intravenous administration of vancomycin, 1.0 gm, over 1 h plus intravenous or intramuscular administration of gentamycin, 1.5 mg/kg (not to exceed 80 mg), 1 h before procedure; may be repeated once 8 h after initial dose
Alternate Low-Risk Patient Regimen	
Amoxicillin	3.0 gm orally 1 h before procedure, then 1.5 gm 6 h after initial dose

* Initial pediatric doses are as follows: ampicillin, 50 mg/kg; amoxicillin, 50 mg/kg; gentamicin, 2.0 mg/kg; and vancomycin, 20 mg/kg. Follow-up doses should be one half of the initial dose. Total pediatric dose should not exceed total adult dose.

Reproduced with permission from reference 9.

Preoperative Considerations

Anesthesia Equipment

FDA Anesthesia Apparatus Checkout Recommendations

This checkout, or a reasonable equivalent, should be conducted before administration of anesthesia. These recommendations are only valid for an anesthesia system that conforms to current and relevant standards and includes an ascending bellows ventilator and at least the following monitors: capnograph, pulse oximeter, oxygen analyzer, respiratory volume monitor (spirometer) and breathing system pressure monitor with high and low pressure alarms.

This is a guidelines which users are encouraged to modify to accommodate differences in equipment design and variations in local clinical practice. Such local modifications should have appropriate peer review. Users should refer to the operator's manual for the manufacturer's specific procedures and precautions, especially the manufacturer's low pressure leak test (step #5).

Emergency Ventilation Equipment

***1. Verify Backup Ventilation Equipment is Available & Functioning**

High Pressure System

***2. Check Oxygen Cylinder Supply**

a. Open O_2 cylinder and verify at least half full (about 1000 psi).
b. Close cylinder.

***3. Check Central Pipeline Supplies**

a. Check that hoses are connected and pipeline gauges read about 50 psi.

Low Pressure System

***4. Check Initial Status of Low Pressure System**

a. Close flow control valves and turn vaporizers off.
b. Check fill level and tighten vaporizers' filler caps.

***5. Perform Leak Check of Machine Low Pressure System**

a. Verify that the machine master switch and flow control valves are OFF.
b. Attach "Suction Bulb" to common (fresh) gas outlet.
c. Squeeze bulb repeatedly until fully collapsed.
d. Verify bulb stays fully collapsed for at least 10 seconds.
e. Open one vaporizer at a time and repeat 'c' and 'd' as above.
f. Remove suction bulb, and reconnect fresh gas hose.

***6. Turn On Machine Master Switch and all other necessary electrical equipment.**

***7. Test Flowmeters**

a. Adjust flow of all gases through their full range, checking for smooth operation of floats and undamaged flowtubes.
b. Attempt to create a hypoxic O_2/N_2O mixture and verify correct changes in flow and/or alarm.

Scavenging System

***8. Adjust and Check Scavenging System**

a. Ensure proper connections between the scavenging system and both APL (pop-off) valve and ventilator relief valve.
b. Adjust waste gas vacuum (if possible).
c. Fully open APL valve and occlude Y-piece.
d. With minimum O_2 flow, allow scavenger reservoir bag to collapse completely and verify that absorber pressure gauge reads about zero.
e. With the O_2 flush activated allow the scavenger reservoir bag to distend fully, and then verify that absorber pressure gauge reads < 10 cm-H_2O.

Breathing System

***9. Calibrate O_2 Monitor**

a. Ensure monitor reads 21% in room air.
b. Verify low O_2 alarm is enabled and functioning.
c. Reinstall sensor in circuit and flush breathing system with O_2.
d. Verify that monitor now reads greater than 90%.

10. Check Initial Status of Breathing System

a. Set selector switch to "Bag" mode.
b. Check that breathing circuit is complete, undamaged and unobstructed.
c. Verify that CO_2 absorbent is adequate.
d. Install breathing circuit accessory equipment (e.g. humidifier, PEEP valve) to be used during the case.

11. Perform Leak Check of the Breathing System

a. Set all gas flows to zero (or minimum).
b. Close APL (pop-off) valve and occlude Y-piece.
c. Pressurize breathing system to about 30 cm H_2O with O_2 flush
d. Ensure that pressure remains fixed for at least 10 seconds.
e. Open APL (pop-off) valve and ensure that pressure decreases.

Manual and Automatic Ventilation Systems

12. Test Ventilation Systems and Unidirectional Valves

a. Place a second breathing bag on Y-piece.
b. Set appropriate ventilator parameters for next patient.
c. Switch to automatic ventilation (Ventilator) mode.
d. Fill bellows and breathing bag with O_2 flush and then turn ventilator ON.
e. Set O_2 flow to minimum, other gas flows to zero.
f. Verify that during inspiration bellows delivers appropriate tidal volume and that during expiration bellows fills completely.
g. Set fresh gas flow to about 5 L/min.
h. Verify that the ventilator bellows and simulated lungs fill, _and empty_ appropriately without sustained pressure at end expiration.
i. _Check for proper action of unidirectional valves._
j. Exercise breathing circuit accessories to ensure proper function.

k. Turn ventilator OFF and switch to manual ventilation (Bag/APL) mode.
l. Ventilate manually and assure inflation and deflation of artificial lungs and appropriate feel of system resistance and compliance.
m. Remove second breathing bag from Y-piece.

Monitors

13. Check, Calibrate and/or Set Alarm Limits of all Monitors

- Capnometer
- Oxygen Analyzer
- Respiratory Volume Monitor (Spirometer)
- Pressure Monitor with High and Low Airway Alarms
- Pulse Oximeter

Final Position

14. Check Final Status of Machine

a. Vaporizers off
b. APL valve open
c. Selector switch to "Bag"
d. All flowmeters to zero
e. Patient suction level adequate
f. Breathing system ready to use

*If an anesthesia provider uses the same machine in successive cases, these steps need not be repeated or may be abbreviated after the initial checkout.

Reprinted with permission from reference 10.

Causes of Failure to Deliver Oxygen to the Alveoli

Upstream of the machine

Liquid oxygen reservoir empty or filled with hypoxic gas (e.g., nitrogen)

Crossed hospital pipelines

Crossed hoses or adapters in the operating room

Closed pipeline valves

Disconnected oxygen hose

Failure of back-up hospital oxygen reserve

Within the machine or circuit

Cylinder filled with hypoxic gas

Empty oxygen cylinder

Incorrect cylinder on oxygen yoke

Crossed pipes within machine

Closed oxygen cylinder valve

Oxygen flowmeter off

Failure of proportioning system

Oxygen leak within the machine or flowmeter

Incompetent or absent circuit unidirectional valves

Breathing circuit leak

Closed system anesthesia with inadequate fresh oxygen supply
Inadequate ventilation

Reprinted with permission from reference 11.

Properties of Commonly Used Medical Gases

	Molecular Weight	Atmospheric Fraction	Density (gm/l)	Specific Gravity (Air = 1)	Solubility Vol % in Water 20°C
Air	28.95	1.0	1.293	1.0	--
Carbon Dioxide	44	0.0004	1.964	1.53	88.0
Helium	4	0.0001	0.178	0.13	0.90
Nitrogen	28	0.7806	1.250	0.96	1.60
Nitrous Oxide	44	--	1.970	1.52	0.63
Oxygen	32	0.2093	1.429	1.11	3.13

Medical Gas Cylinders Color Code

Gas	Formula	Color (USA)	Color (International)	Pressure (psi at 21°C)	State in Cylinder	Capacity of E Cylinder (L)
Oxygen	O_2	Green	White	1900 - 2200	Gas	660
Carbon Dioxide	CO_2	Gray	Gray	838	Liquid < 31°C	1590
Nitrous Oxide	N_2O	Blue	Blue	745	Liquid < 37°C	1600
Cyclopropane	C_3H_6	Orange	Orange	75	Liquid	1440
Helium	He	Brown	Brown	1600 - 2000	Gas	500
Nitrogen	N_2	Black	Black	1800 - 2200	Gas	660
Air		Yellow‡	Black & White	1800	Gas	600

‡Air, including mixtures of oxygen with nitrogen containing 19.5 - 23.5% oxygen, is color-coded yellow. Mixtures of nitrogen and oxygen other than those containing 19.5 - 23.5% oxygen are color-coded black and green.

Modified with permission from reference 12.

Typical Medical Gas Cylinders

Cylinder Dimensions	Capacity	Carbon dioxide	Cyclo-propane	Helium	Nitrous Oxide	Oxygen	Helium-Oxygen Mixtures	CO_2 Oxygen Mixtures	Wt (lb) Empty Cylinder
A (3" o.d. x 7")	Lb	0.8	0.6	0.02	0.8	0.23			
	Liters	189	151	57	189	76	57	76	3
	Gal	50	40	15	50	20	15	20	
B (3.5" o.d. x 13")	Lb	1.6	1.5	0.06	1.5	0.6			
	Liters	378	378	148	378	196	113	150	6
	Gal	100	100	39	100	52	40	40	
D (4.25" o.d. x 17")	Lb	3.8	3.3	0.1	3.8	1.2			
	Liters	946	871	299	946	396	299	396	10
	Gal	250	230	79	250	105	79	105	
E (4.25" o.d. x 26")	Lb	6.6	5.5	0.2	6.4	1.9			
	Liters	1,590	1,438	496	1,590	659	496	659	13
	Gal	420	380	131	420	174	131	174	
F (5.5" o.d. x 51")	Lb	20		0.6	21.0	6.0			
	Liters	4,800		1,585	5,260	2,062	1,640	2,062	67
	Gal	1,270		420	1,400	545	433	545	
M (7" o.d. x 43")	Lb	30.6		0.9	30.6	8.8			
	Liters	7,570		2,263	7,570	3,000	2,263	3,000	70
	Gal	2,000		598	2,000	800	598	800	

Cylinder Dimensions	Capacity	Carbon dioxide	Cyclo-propane	Helium	Nitrous Oxide	Oxygen	Helium-Oxygen Mixtures	CO_2 Oxygen Mixtures	Wt (lb) Empty Cylinder
G (8.5" o.d. x 51")	Lb	50		1.5	56.0	15.5			
	Liters	12,358		4,016	13,836	5,331	4,016	5,300	110
	Gal	3,260		1,061	3,655	1,408	1,061	1,400	
H & K (9.25" o.d. x 51")	Lb				64.3	16-22			
	Liters				15,899	5,570-7,500			130
	Gal				4,200	1,470-2,000			
AA* (2.75" o.d. x 11")	Lb		0.6						
	Liters		150						3
	Gal		40						
BB* (2.75" o.d. x 19.75")	Lb		1.25						
	Liters		377						4
	Gal		100						
DD* (3.75" o.d. x 23.77")	Lb		3.3						
	Liters		850						8
	Gal		220						

* Chromium-plated cylinders.

Reproduced with permission from reference 12.

Capnography and Capnometry with Altered Carbon Dioxide Production

	Waveform on Capnograph	End-Tidal CO_2	Inspiratory CO_2	End-Tidal to Arterial Gradient
Absorption of carbon dioxide from peritoneal cavity	Normal	↑	0	Normal
Injection of sodium bicarbonate	Normal	↑	0	Normal
Pain, anxiety, shivering	Normal	↑	0	Normal
Increased muscle tone (as from muscle relaxant reversal)	Normal	↑	0	Normal
Convulsions	Normal	↑	0	Normal
Hyperthermia	Normal	↑	0	Normal
Hypothermia	Normal	↓	0	Normal
Increased depth of anesthesia (in relation to surgical stimulus)	Normal	↓	0	Normal
Use of muscle relaxants	May see curare cleft	↓	0	Normal

Normal end-tidal carbon dioxide is 38 torr (5%). Inspired carbon dioxide is normally 0. The arterial to end-tidal gradient is normally less than 5 torr.

Reproduced with permission from reference 12.

Cagnographic and Capnometric Alterations as a Result of Circulatory Changes

	Waveform on Capnograph	End-Tidal CO_2	Inspired CO_2	End-Tidal to Arterial Gradient
Decreased transport of carbon dioxide to the lungs (impaired peripheral circulation)	Normal	↓	0	Normal
Decreased transport of carbon dioxide through the lungs (pulmonary embolus, either air or thrombus; surgical manipulations)	Normal	↓	0	Elevated
Right to left shunt	Normal	↑	0	Elevated
Increased patient dead space	Normal	↓	0	Elevated
Increased transport of carbon dioxide to the lungs (restoration of peripheral circulation after it has been impaired, e.g., after release of a tourniquet)	Normal	↑	0	Normal

Reproduced with permission from reference 12.

Capnometry and Capnography with Respiratory Problems

	Waveform on Capnograph	End-Tidal CO_2	Inspiratory CO_2	End-Tidal to Alveolar Gradient
Disconnection	Absent		0	
Apneic patient, stopped ventilator	Absent		0	
Endobronchial incubation	May show sloping ascending limb	↑	0	Elevated
Hyperventilation	Normal	↓	0	Normal
Hypoventilation, mild to moderate	Normal	↑	0	Normal
Hypoventilation, extreme	Abnormal	↓	0	Elevated
Upper airway obstruction	Abnormal	↑	0	Elevated
Rebreathing (e.g, under drapes)	Baseline elevated	↑	↑	Normal
Esophageal intubation	Absent		0	

Reproduced with permission from reference 12.

Capnographic and Capnometric Alterations Seen with Equipment Problems

	Waveform on Capnograph	End-Tidal CO_2	Inspired CO_2	Arterial to End-Tidal Gradient
Increased apparatus dead space	Baseline Elevated	↑	↑	Normal
Circle system: Faulty unidirectional valve, faulty or exhausted absorbent, bypassed absorber	Baseline Elevated	↑	↑	Normal
Inadequate fresh gas flow to a Mapleson system	Baseline	↑	↑	Normal
	Elevated	↑		
Problems with the inner tube of a Bain system	Baseline	↑	↑	Normal
	Elevated	↑		
Malfunctioning non-rebreathing valve with rebreathing	Baseline Elevated	↑	↑	Normal
Obstruction to expiration in the breathing system	Abnormal	↑	0	Elevated
Leakage in breathing system	Abnormal	↓	0	Elevated
Water in sampling cell	Abnormal	↑	↑	Elevated
Water blocking sampling line	Absent			
Leakage in sampling line	Abnormal	↓	0	Elevated
Too low a flow rate with aspiration devices	Abnormal	↓	↑	Elevated
Too high a flow rate with aspiration devices	Abnormal	↓	0	↑
Inadequate seal around endotracheal tube	Abnormal	↓	0	↑

Reproduced with permission from reference 12.

Mapleson Classification of Rebreathing Systems A Through F

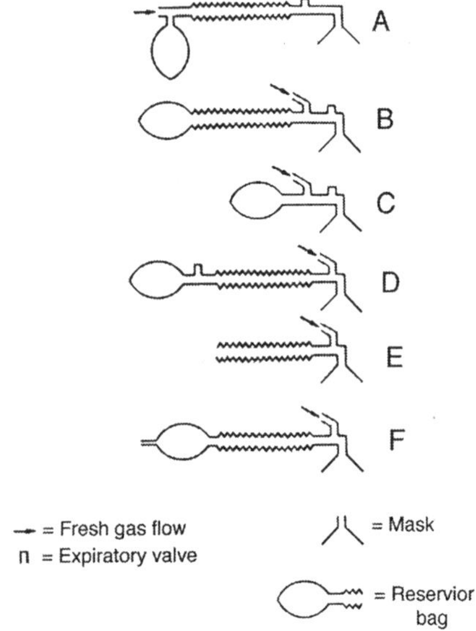

Reproduced with permission from reference 13.

Bain Circuit. Coaxial Mapleson D.

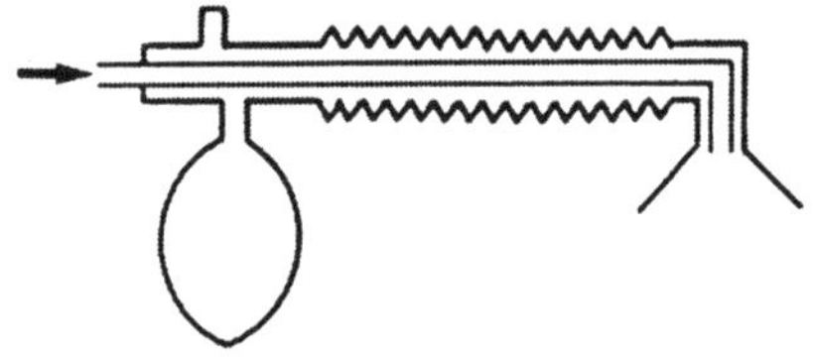

Arrow indicates fresh gasflow.

Reproduced with permission from reference 11.

Indicators for Carbon Dioxide Absorbents

Indicator	Color when Fresh	Color when Exhausted
Phenolphthalein	White	Pink
Ethyl violet	White	Purple
Clayton Yellow	Red	Yellow
Ethyl Orange	Orange	Yellow
Mimosa Z	Red	White

Reproduced from reference 12.

Commonly Available Blood Pressure Cuffs

Cuff Name*	Bladder Width (cm)	Bladder Length (cm)
Newborn	2.5 - 4.0	5.0 - 9.0
Infant	4.0 - 6.0	11.5 - 18.0
Child	7.5 - 9.0	17.0 - 19.0
Adult	11.5 - 13.0	22.0 - 26.0
Large arm	14.0 - 15.0	30.5 - 33.0
Thigh	18.0 - 19.0	36.0 - 38.0

* Cuff name does not guarantee that the cuff will be an appropriate size for a child within that age range.

Reproduced with permission from reference 14.

Sites of Neurostimulation

Nerve	Location	Movement observed
Ulnar	Wrist or elbow	Thumb adduction, flexion of fourth and fifth fingers, abduction of fifth finger
Posterior tibial	Posterior to the medial malleolus	Plantar flexion of the big toe
Peroneal	Lateral to the neck of the fibula	Dorsiflexion of the foot
Facial	Near the tragus where the nerve emerges from the stylomastoid foremen, 2 to 3 cm posterior to the orbit	Contraction of orbicularis oculi or obicularis oris

Reprinted with permission from reference 11.

Approximate Relationships Among Percent Receptor Block, Single-Twitch, and Train-of-Four During Nondepolarizing Block

Total receptors blocked (% of)	Twitch (T_1) (% normal)	T_4 (% normal)	T_4/T_1
100	0	0	-
90 - 95	0	0	T_1 lost
85 - 90	10	0	T_2 lost
—	20	0	T_3 lost
80 - 85	25	0	T_4 lost
—	80 - 90	48 - 58	0.60 - 0.70
—	95	69 - 79	0.70 - 0.75
75	100	75 - 100	0.75 - 1.0
—	100	100	0.90 - 1.0
50	100	100	1.0
25	100	100	1.0

Reprinted with permission from reference 11.

Lasers Commonly Used in the Operating Room

Laser	Wavelength (nanometers)	General considerations
Argon	488 - 515 (blue/green)	Absorbed selectively by hemoglobin and melanin or other similar pigments Transmitted through clear substances Tissue penetration: 0.5 to 2 mm
KTP* (frequency-doubled YAG)	532 (green)	Strongly absorbed by hemoglobin, melanin, and similar pigments Transmitted through clear substances Tissue penetration: 0.5 to 2 mm
Dye laser	Variable with dyes	Wavelength can be tuned to suit application; e.g., 585 nm (yellow) for hemoglobin absorption and 630 nm (red) for photodynamic therapy
Nd:YAG†	1064 (near infrared)	More readily absorbed by dark tissue Transmitted through clear fluids Tissue penetration: 2 to 6 mm
CO_2	10,600 (far infrared)	Strongly absorbed by water and thus by all tissue, pigmented or not Tissue penetration: <0.5 mm
He-Ne‡	633 (red)	Used as a low-power coaxial aiming beam for nonvisible lasers (CO_2 and Nd:YAG) Has no significant tissue interaction

*Potassium titanyl phosphate
†Neodymium-doped yttrium-aluminum-garnet
‡Helium-neon.

Reproduced with permission from reference 11.

Generic Pacemaker Code

I Chamber(s) Paced	II Chamber(s) Sensed	III Modes of Response(s)	IV Programmable Functions	V Special Antitachycardia Functions(s)
O = None	O = None	O = None	O = None	O = None
A = Atrium	A = Atrium	I = Inhibited	P = Simple Programmable (rate and/or output)	P = Pacing (antitachyarrhythmia)
V = Ventricle	V = Ventricle	T = Triggered	M = Multiprogrammable	S = Shock
D = Dual (A + V)	D = Dual	D = Dual (T + I)*	C = Communicating	D = Dual (P + S)

*Atrial triggered and ventricular inhibited.

Generic Codes for Single- and Dual-Chamber Pacing Modalities

AOO, VOO, DOO	Atrial asynchronous, ventricular asynchronous, or dual-sequential asynchronous pacing
AAI, VVI, DVI	Atrial-inhibited, ventricular-inhibited, or dual-sequential ventricular-inhibited pacing
VAT or VDD	Atrial-triggered ventricular, or atrial-triggered, ventricular-inhibited pacing
DDI or DDD	Dual-sequential, atrial-ventricular-inhibited, or dual-sequential, atrial-triggered-ventricular inhibited pacing

Reproduced with permission from reference 7.

Available Pacemaker Modalities, Function, and Applications

Type	Function	Applications
Asynchronous	Paces atria (AOO) or ventricles (VOO)	Temporary pacing of atria (with intact AV conduction) or ventricles for bradycardia
Synchronous	Both paces and senses atria (AAI, CAT) or ventricles (VVI, VVT), with sensing circuit either inhibiting (I) or triggering (T) the pacing circuit	Temporary or permanent pacing of atria or ventricles in patients with bradycardia and/or AV conduction block
AV sequential	Paces atria or ventricles and senses ventricle (DVI), or paces and senses both atria and ventricles (DDD); preserves the atrioventricular contraction sequence	Temporary or permanent pacing in critically ill patients for bradycardia with heart block, but who also need the atrial contribution to ventricular filling
Programmable	Programs rate, stimulus output, R- and P-wave sensitivity, refractory periods, P-R intervals, synchronous and asynchronous functions, and hysteresis (whereby pacemaker is inhibited over wide range of normal sinus rates)	Permanent pacemakers only; optimizes pacemaker function or specific or changing patient needs; minimizes the need for invasive procedures to correct malfunction

Reproduced with permission from reference 15.

Customary Uses for Four Available Temporary Cardiac Pacing Routes

Epicardial

Atrial, ventricular, sequential pacing

Cardiac surgery following sternotomy

Usually preferred in infants and children

Transvenous

Atrial, ventricular, sequential pacing

Entended pacing in conscious patients

Before elective pacemaker implantation

Transcutaneous

Initial pacing with brady-systolic arrest

Bradycardia with atrial fibrillation*

Bradycardia with third-degree AV heart bolck*

Transesophageal

Initial pacing with intact AV conduction*

Transient perioperative brady arrhythmias†

Prophylaxis for sinus node dysfunction

*Until venous or epicardial pacing can be established.
†Provided the patient is not in atrial fibrillation.

Reprinted with permission from reference 7.

Macroshock and Microshock Hazards

Effects of 60-Hz AC on an Average Human for a 1-Second Duration of Contact

Current	Effect
Macroshock	
1 mA (0.001 A)	Threshold of perception
5 mA (0.005 A)	Accepted as maximum harmless current intensity
10 - 20 mA (0.01-0.02 A)	"Let-go" current before sustained muscle contraction
50 mA (0.05 A)	Pain, possible fainting, mechanical injury; heart and respiratory functions continue
100-300 mA (0.1-0.3 A)	Ventricular fibrillation will start, but respiratory center remains intact
6000 mA (6 A)	Sustained myocardial contractions, followed by normal heart rhythm; temporary respiratory paralysis; burns if current density is high
Microshock	
100 μA (0.1 mA)	Ventricular fibrillation
10 μA (0.01 mA)	Recommended maximum allowable 60-Hz leakage current

A = amperes; mA = millamperes; μA = microamperes.

Reproduced with permission from reference 11.

Needle Sizes / Catheter Sizes

Outer Diameter Conversions

Gauge	French	Inches	Millimeters
-	0.79	0.010	0.26
-	1.00	0.013	0.33
-	1.08	0.014	0.36
27	1.23	0.016	0.41
26	1.36	0.018	0.46
25	1.52	0.020	0.51
24	1.68	0.022	0.56
23	1.92	0.025	0.64
22	2.13	0.028	0.71
21	2.43	0.032	0.82
20	2.69	0.035	0.90
-	2.92	0.038	0.97
-	3.00	0.039	1.00
19	3.20	0.042	1.07
18	3.77	0.049	1.26
-	4.00	0.053	1.35
17	4.42	0.058	1.47
16	5.00	0.066	1.67
15	5.50	0.072	1.83
-	6.00	0.079	2.00
14	6.50	0.083	2.17
-	7.00	0.092	2.30
13	7.24	0.095	2.41
-	8.00	0.105	2.70
-	9.00	0.118	3.00
-	10.00	0.131	3.30
-	11.00	0.144	3.77
-	12.00	0.168	4.00
-	14.00	0.184	4.70
-	16.00	0.210	5.30
-	18.00	0.236	6.00
-	20.00	0.263	6.70
-	22.00	0.288	7.30

French size = (outer diameter in mm) x 3

Pharmacology

Inhalational Anesthetics

Properties of Volatile Anesthetic Agents

	Halothane	Enflurane	Isoflurane	Sevoflurane	Desflurane
Odor	Sweet, non-pungent	Mildly pungent, ethereal	Markedly pungent, ethereal	Minimally pungent	Markedly pungent ethereal
Blood/gas partition coefficient:					
Adults	2.3	1.9	1.4	0.7	0.4
Neonates	2.1	1.8	1.2	0.7	
MAC (%):					
Adults	0.8	1.7	1.2	2.0	6.0
Neonates	0.9	2.4	1.6	3.3	9.2
Rate of metabolism (%)	20.0	2.0	0.2	2.0	0.02
Myocardial depression	++	+++	+	?+	+
Peripheral vasodilatation	+	+	++	?++	++
Respiratory depression	+	+++	++	++	++

Adapted with permission from reference 15.

Table of Inhalational Anesthetic Physical Constants

Generic Name	Brand Name	Structural Formula	Mol. Weight	Density g/ml (°C)	Boiling Point (°C)	Vapor Press (°C)	Water: Gas	Blood: Gas	Oil: Gas	Human MAC	Animal MAC
Isoflurane	Forane	$CF_3\text{-}CHCl\text{-}O\text{-}CHF_2$	184.5	1.496 (25)	48.5	238.1 (20) 488.83 (37)	0.606	1.407	97.8	1.15	1.46
Enflurane	Ethrane	$CFHCl\text{-}CF_2\text{-}O\text{-}CHF_2$	184.5	1.518 (25)	56.5	174.5 (20) 345.2 (36)	0.82	1.91	98.2	1.7	2.2
Halothane	Fluothane	$CF_3\text{-}CHClBr$	197.41	1.874 (20)	50.2	243 (20) 487 (37)	0.74	2.3	224	0.75	0.87
Sevoflurane	Ultane	$CH(CF_3)_2\text{-}O\text{-}CH_2F$	200.06	1.505	58.5	160 (20) 200 (25) 317 (37)	0.37	0.686	47.2	1.7 - 2.1	2.5
Desflurane	Suprane	$CF_3\text{-}CHF\text{-}O\text{-}CHF_2$	168.0	1.451 (20)	23.5	664 (20)	0.225	0.424	18.7	6.0	5.7
Methoxyflurane	Penthrane	$CHCl_2\text{-}CF_2\text{-}O\text{-}CH_3$	164.98	1.431 (20)	104.65	23 (20) 56 (37)	4.5	13.0	825	0.16	0.23
Nitrous Oxide		$N \equiv N = O$	44.01	1.997 (0)	-88.5	59300 (37)	0.435	0.468	1.4	1.05*	1.47*
Diethyl Ether	Ether	$CH_3\text{-}CH_2\text{-}O\text{-}CH_2\text{-}CH_3$	74.12	0.714 (20)	34.6	442.2 (20) 820 (37)	13.09	12.1	656	1.9	3.04

*Indicates atmospheres, rather than volume percent

Volatile Anesthetic Concentrations

$\%$ anesthetic $= 100\ V_A / V_t = 100\ (P_v)VO_{2vap} / V_t(P_b\text{-}P_v) = 100\ (VO_{2vap})\ P_v / (VO_{2vap})\ (Pb) + (V_{dil})\ (Pb\text{-}P_v)$

where:

V_A = anesthetic vapor output in ml/min
V_t = total gas flow in ml/min
Pv = vapor pressure of volatile anesthetic
VO_{2vap} = O_2 passing through vaporizer in ml/min
Pb = barometric pressure
V_{dil} = volume of diluent gases in ml/min

Output in Per Cent and MAC in O_2 of Erroneously Filled Vaporizers at 22 °C

Vaporizers	Liquid	Setting %	Output%	Output MAC
Halothane	Halothane	1.0	1.00	1.25
	Enflurane	1.0	0.62	0.37
	Isoflurane	1.0	0.96	0.84
Enflurane	Enflurane	2.0	2.00	1.19
	Isoflurane	2.0	3.09	2.69
	Halothane	2.0	3.21	4.01
Isoflurane	Isoflurane	1.5	1.50	1.30
	Halothane	1.5	1.56	1.95
	Enflurane	1.5	0.97	0.57

Reprinted with permission from reference 16.

Vaporizer Output after Incorrectly Refilling from 25% Full to 100% Full

			Vaporizer Outputs						
			Halothane		Enflurane		Isoflurane		
Vaporizer	Setting %	Refill Liquid	%	MAC	%	MAC	%	MAC	Total MAC
Halothane	1.0	Enflurane	0.33	0.41	0.64	0.38	—	—	0.79
	1.0	Isoflurane	0.41	0.51	—	—	0.90	0.78	1.29
Enflurane	2.0	Halothane	2.43	3.03	0.96	0.57	—	—	3.60
Isoflurane	I.5	Halothane	1.28	1.60	—	—	0.57	0.50	2.10

Reprinted with permission from reference 16.

Cardiovascular Effects of Selected Volatile Anesthetics

	Enflurane	Halothane	Isoflurane
Heart Rate	O / ↑	O / ↓	↑↑
Blood Pressure	↓↓	↓↓	↓↓
Cardiac Output	↓↓	↓↓	O - ↑
Cardiac Contraction	↓↓↓	↓↓	↓ - ↓↓
Vascular Resistance	O - ↓	O	↓↓
Central Venous Pressure	↑	↑	O
Sensitization of the Heart to Epinephrine	↑	↑↑↑	↑↑

Pharmacology

Narcotics and Other Pain Medications

Classification of Opioid Agonists and Antagonists

Opioid agonists	Opioid agonist-antagonists	Opioid antagonists
Morphine	Pentazocine (Talwin)	Naloxone (Narcan)
Meperidine (Demerol)	Nalorphine (Nalline)	Naltrexone (Trexan)
Fentanyl (Sublimaze)	Butorphanol (Stadol)	Nalmefene (Revex)
Sufentanil (Sufenta)	Nalbuphine (Nubain)	
Alfentanil (Alfenta)	Buprenorphine (Buprenex)*	
Codeine	Dezocine (Dalgan)	
Dextromethorphan		
Hydromorphone (Dilaudid)		
Oxymorphone (Numorphan)		
Methadone (Dolophine)		
Heroin		

*Partial agonist.

Modified with permission from reference 18.

Opioid Analgesics And Antagonists

Drug and Year of Introduction	Protein Binding (%)	Half-Life (hr)	Receptors & Effects	Equiv Dose to Morph (10 mg IM)	Route	Dose (mg)	Onset (min)	Duration (hr)	Metabolism Comments
Agonists									
Alfentanil 1986	92	1.5	mu+	0.3	IV	3.5 - 8.5	rapid	0.2 - 0.3	met - liver
Codeine 1832	<10	2.5 - 4	-	120	PO IM, SC	15 - 60 15 - 60	30 - 40 10 - 30	4 4	met - liver
Fentanyl (Sublimaze) 1968	65 - 90	1 - 4	mu+	0.1	IM IV	0.05 - 0.1 0.025 - 0.1	7 - 15 rapid	1 - 2 0.5 - 1	met - liver larger doses used in anesthesia; very large doses (7 mg) prolong duration (24 - 36 hr)
Hydrocodone (Hycodan) 1943	--	3.8	--	5 - 10	PO	5 - 10	10 - 30	4 - 6	met - liver
Hydromorphone (Dilaudid) 1926	20 - 40	2.6 - 4	--	2	PO, IM, SC IV PR	2 - 4 3 - 4 3	15 - 30 10 10 - 15	4 2 - 4 6 - 8	met - liver, primarily
Meperidine Pethidine (Demerol) 1939	60	2.4 - 4	mu+ kappa+	120	PO, IM, SC IV	50 - 150 50 - 150	10 - 15 1	2 - 4 2 - 4	met - liver, active metabolites hyperthermic crisis with MAOIs; prolonged by renal failure

Drug and Year of Introduction	Protein Binding (%)	Half-Life (hr)	Receptors and Effects	Equivalent Dose to Morphine (10 mg IM)	Route	Dose (mg)	Onset (min)	Duration (hr)	Metabolism Comments
Methadone (Dolophine) 1943	85	15 - 25	mu+	8	PO IM	2.5 - 20 2.5 - 20	30 - 60 10 - 20	4 - 6 4 - 6	met - liver beware accumulation due to long half-life
Morphine 1806	10 - 34	2 - 3	mu+ kappa+	10	PO IM, IV, SC	10 - 30 2.5 - 10	10 - 30 10 - 30	4 - 5 4 - 5	met - liver significant histamine release
Oxymorphone (Numorphan) 1959	--	3 - 6	mu+ kappa+ delta+ sigma	1	IM, IV, SC	0.5 - 1.5	5 - 20	3 - 6	met - liver
Oxycodone (Percodan) 1950	--	2.8 - 3.5	--	--	PO	3 - 5	30 - 45	6	met - liver
Propoxyphene (Darvon) 1957	65 - 90	6 - 12	mu+ kappa+ sigma+	180 - 240	PO	65	15 - 60	4 - 6	met - liver variable effectiveness as an analgesic
Sufentanil (Sufenta) 1984	92.5	2.5	mu+	0.01	IV	0.01 - 0.025	rapid	0.5 - 1	met - liver, small intestine large doses used in anesthesia prolong recovery

Drug and Year of Introduction	Protein Binding (%)	Half-Life (hr)	Receptors and Effects	Equivalent Dose to Morphine (10 mg IM)	Route	Dose (mg)	Onset (min)	Duration (hr)	Metabolism Comments
Agonists-Antagonists									
Buprenorphine (Buprenex) 1985	96	3	mu p	0.4	PO, IM IV, SC	0.3 - 0.6	5	6	met - liver (minimal)
Butorphanol (Stadol) 1978	65 - 90	2.5 - 4	kappa+ sigma+	2	IM IV	1 - 4 0.5 - 2	10 - 30 2 - 3	3 - 4 3 - 4	met - liver
Nalbuphine (Nubain) 1979	60 - 70	3 - 6	mu- kappa p sigma	10	IM, SC IV	0.15 0.15	10 - 15 2 - 3	3 - 6 3 - 6	met - liver
Pentazocine (Talwin) 1967	35 - 64	2 - 3	mu- kappa+ sigma	60	PO IM, SC IV	50 30 30	15 - 30 15 - 20 2 - 3	3 2 - 3 2 - 3	met - liver
Antagonists									
Naloxone (Narcan) 1971	46	0.5 - 1.3	mu- kappa- delta- sigma	--	IM, IV SC	0.4 - 0.8	2 - 5	1 - 4	met - liver used in smaller doses postop, titrated to achieve adequate ventilation
Naltrexone (Trexan) 1984	21	4 - 10	mu- kappa- delta- sigma	--	PO	100	120 - 180	48	met - liver used to maintain opioid avoidance in previous addicts

Receptor: + = agonist; p = partial agonist; - = antagonist.

Reprinted with permission from reference 19.

Opioid Analgesics And Antagonists Equivalent Doses

Equivalent Dose to Morphine (10 mg IM)	mg
Sufentanil	0.01
Fentanyl	0.1
Alfentanil	0.3
Buprenorphine	0.4
Oxymorphone	1
Butorphanol	2
Hydromorphone	2
Hydrocodone	5 - 10
Methadone	8
Morphine	10
Nalbuphine	10
Pentazocine	60
Codeine	120
Meperidine	120
Propoxyphene	180 - 240

Epidural Opioid Doses

Drug	Dose (mg)	Onset (min)	Duration (hr)
Alfentanil	2	5	1
Sufentanil	0.005 - 0.010	3 - 5	2 - 4
Fentanyl	0.05 - 0.10	5 - 20	3 - 5
Methadone	5 - 8	10 - 20	6 - 8
Hydromorphone	1	15 - 20	7 - 15
Meperidine	30 - 100	5 - 10	4 - 20
Morphine	3 - 5	30 - 60	12 - 24

Nonnarcotic Analgesics for Children

Drug	Dose	Interval	Route*
Ibuprofen	4 - 10 mg/kg	q 6 - 8 h	PO
Naproxen (Naprosyn, Syntex)	5 - 7 mg/kg	q 6 - 8 h	PO
Tolmetin (Tolectin, McNeil)	5 - 7 mg/kg	q 6 - 8 h	PO
Choline magnesium salicylate (Trilisate, Purdue Frederick)	10 - 15 mg/kg	q 8 h	PO
Ketorolac tromethamine (Toradol, Syntex)	First dose: 1 mg/kg Repeat doses: 0.5 mg/kg	q 6 h	IV or IM
Acetaminophen	10 - 15 mg/kg 15 - 20 mg/kg	q 4h q 4 h	PO PR

*PO = by mouth; PR = per rectum; IV = intravenous; IM = intramuscular.

Reprinted with permission from reference 20.

Pharmacology of Opioid Receptors

	Mu (μ)				
Receptor	μ_1	μ_2	**Delta** (δ)	**Kappa** (K)	**Sigma** (σ)
Effect					
Analgesia	Supraspinal*		Spinal	Spinal	
Affect	Euphoria	Sedation		Sedation	Dysphoria/ Hallucinations
Pupil	Miosis			Miosis	Mydriasis
Respiration		Depression	Depression		Tachypnea
Gastrointestinal	Nausea/ Vomiting	Constipation	Nausea/ Vomiting		
Genitourinary	Urinary/ Retention		Urinary/ Retention	Diuresis	
Temperature	Increase				
Other	Pruritus		Pruritus Physical Dependence		
Tolerance	Yes		Yes	Little	
Cross Tolerance	δ		μ	No	

* Includes periaqueductal nucleus raphe magnus and locus coeruleus

Receptor	**Mu** (μ)		**Delta** (δ)		**Kappa** (Κ)		**Sigma** (σ)	
Binding Properties	Affinity	Activity	Affinity	Activity	Affinity	Activity	Affinity	Activity
Agonists								
Morphine	+++	+++	++	++	+	+		
Meperidine	++	++	++	++	+	+		
Fentanyl	++++	++++	+	+				
Agonist-Antagonists								
Pentazocine	++	0			+++	+++	+++	+++
Nalbuphine	++	0			+++	+++	++	+
Butorphanol	++	0			+++	++	++	++
Buprenorphine	+++	+			++			
Dezocine	+++	+	++	+	+	+		

Key: Affinity: + low affinity, ++ moderate affinity, +++ high affinity, ++++ very high affinity.
Activity: 0 no activity, + low activity, + + moderate activity, + + + high activity, + + + + very high activity.

Adapted with permission from reference 21.

Nonsteroidal Anti-Inflammatory Agents, by Classes

Acidic agents

Carboxylic acids

Salicylates
- Aspirin
- Lysine acetyl salicylate
- Choline magnesium trisalicylate
- Salsalate
- Magnesium salicylate
- Lithium salicylate*
- Imidazole salicylate

Difluorophenyl derivative
- Diflunisal

Fenamates
- Meclofenamate
- Mefenamic acid
- Flufenamic acid
- Tolfenamic acid

Pyranocarboxylic acid
- Etodolac

Alkanoic acids

Propionic acids
- Ibuprofen
- Naproxen
- Fenoprofen
- Indoprofen*
- Suprofen*
- Tiaprofenic acid
- Protizinic acid
- Pirprofen
- Flurbiprofen
- Carprofen
- Benoxaprofen*
- Ketoprofen

Indoleacetic acids
- Indomethacin
- Sulindac

Aryl acetic acids
- Alclofenac*
- Diclofenac
- Fenclofenac

Heteroaryl acetic acids
- Tolmetin
- Zomepirac*
- Ketorolac

Enolic acids

Oxicams
- Piroxicam
- Tenoxicam

Pyrazolidinediones
- Phenylbutazone
- Oxyphenbutazone*
- Azapropazone

Nonacidic agents

p-Aminophenols
- Acetaminophen
- Phenacetin*

Pyrazoles
- Dipyrone

Naphthylalkanone
- Nabumetone

*Withdrawn because of toxicity.

Reprinted with permission from reference 22.

NSAIDs Maximum Daily Doses and Dosage Forms (Available in the United States)

Agents		Maximum Adult dose (24 hours)	t_{peak} (hours)	$t_{1/2}$ (hours)	Dosage interval (hours)
Salicylates					
Aspirin	e, rs*	3.6 - 7.2 g	0.5 - 2	2 - 30	4
Choline salicylate (Arthropan)	e	4.8 - 7.2 g	0.5 - 2	2 - 30	4
Choline magnesium trisalicylate (Trilisate)	e	3 g	1 - 2	9 - 17	8 - 24
Sodium salicylate (Pabalate, etc.)	i	3.6 - 5.4 g	0.5 - 2	2 - 30	4
Salsalate (Disalcid)		3 - 4 g	2 - 4	16	6 - 12
Propionic acids					
Ibuprofen (Motrin, etc.)	e	3200 mg	1 - 2	2 - 3	6 - 8
Fenoprofen (Nalfon)		3200 mg	1 - 2	2 - 3	4 - 6
Ketoprofen (Orudis)		300 mg	1 - 2	2 - 4	6 - 8
Flurbiprofen (Ansaid)	o	300 mg	1 - 5	4 - 6	6 - 8
Naproxen (Naprosyn)	e	1500 mg	2 - 4	12 - 15	12
Naproxen sodium (Anaprox)		1375 mg	1 - 2	13	6 - 8

Agents		Maximum Adult dose (24 hours)	t_{peak} (hours)	$t_{1/2}$ (hours)	Dosage interval (hours)
Fenamates					
Meclofenamate (Meclomen)		400 mg	0.5 - 1	2 - 3	6 - 8
Mefenamic acid (Ponstel)		1000 mg	2 - 4	2 - 4	6
Oxicams					
Piroxicam (Feldene)		20 mg	3 - 5	50	24
Acetic acids					
Indomethacin (Indocin)	rs, i	200 mg	1 - 3	2 - 5	4 - 12
Sulindac (Clinoril)		400 mg	2 - 4	8 - 18	12
Tolmetin (Tolectin)		2000 mg	0.5 - 1	1 - 5	6 - 8
Etodolac (Lodine)		1200 mg	1 - 2	7	6 - 12
Diclofenac (Voltaren)		200 mg	1 - 3	1 - 2	6
Ketorolac (Toradol)		60 mg (oral)	0.5 - 1	4 - 9	6
	i	120-150 mg(IM)			
Nonacidic agents					
Acetaminophen	e, re	4 g	0.5 - 1	1 - 4	4
Nabumetone (Relafen)		1000 mg	3 - 6	24	12 - 2 4

*Alternative dose forms available in the United States; rs = rectal suppository, e = elixir, o = ophthalmic, i = injectable.

Reprinted with permission from reference 22.

Opiates in Common Use in Pediatric/Neonate ICUs

Drug	Route of administration	Starting dose*,†	Duration (hours)
Morphine	Intermittent IV	0.05 - 0.1 mg/kg	2 - 4
	Continuous IV	0.01 - 0.1 mg/kg/h	N/A
	Intramuscular	0.1 - 0.15 mg/kg	3 - 4
	Oral	3 mg/kg	3 - 4
Meperidine	Intermittent IV	0.8 - 1.0 mg/kg	2 - 4
	Continuous IV	0.3 - 0.6 mg/kg/h	NA
	Intramuscular	1 - 1.5 mg/kg	3 - 4
	Oral	1 - 2 mg/kg	4
Fentanyl	Intermittent IV	1 - 2 μg/kg	1 - 2
	Continuous IV	1 - 2 μg/kg/h	NA
Methadone	Intermittent IV	0.05 - 0.1 mg/kg	4 - 12
	Oral	0.1 - 0.15 mg/kg	4 - 8
Codeine	Oral	0.5 - 1.0 mg/kg	4
	Intramuscular	0.5 - 1.0 mg/kg	4

*Use low-dose recommendations in spontaneously ventilating neonates and be prepared for respiratory depression.
†Before starting an infusion of any narcotic, give a loading IV dose of the same narcotic, sufficient to achieve analgesia.

Reprinted with permission from reference 20.

Pharmacology

Barbiturates, Benzodiazepines and Related Drugs

Benzodiazepines

Comparison of Short-Acting Anxiolytics (Benzodiazepines and Hydroxyzine)

Drug and Year of Introduction	Protein Binding (%)	Half-Life (hr)	Solubility	Route	Dose (mg)	Frequency (hr)	Onset (min)	Peak (hr)	Use
Alprazolam (Xanax) 1981	80	12 - 15	lipid-soluble; acid pH increases water solubility	PO	0.25 - 1	8	2 hr	0.7 - 1.2	anxiolytic
Lorazepam (Ativan) 1979	93	10 - 20	water soluble; onset lower IV due to poor lipid solubility	PO IM IV	0.5 - 2 2 - 4 2 - 4	8 - 12 8 - 12 PRN	15 - 45 15 - 30 1 - 5	2 - 5 1 - 1.5 immediate	anxiolytic amne-stic induction agent
Oxazepam (Serax) 1968	95 - 98	5 - 15	water soluble	PO	10 - 30	6 - 8	45 - 90	2 - 4	sedative-hypnotic anxiolytic
Temazepam (Restoril) 1981	96	10 - 20	poorly water soluble	PO	15 - 30	6	45 - 60	2 - 3	sedative-hypnotic

Drug and Year of Introduction	Protein Binding (%)	Half-Life (hr)	Solubility	Route	Dose (mg)	Frequency (hr)	Onset (min)	Peak (hr)	Use
Triazolam (Halcion) 1983	94 - 98	1.7 - 3	poorly water soluble	PO	0.25 - 0.5	8	17 - 18	1 - 3	hypnotic
Hydroxyzine (Atarax, Vistaril) 1958	minimal	8.9	water soluble	PO	50 - 100	6	15 - 30	1 - 2	sedative-hypnotic anxiolytic
				IM	50 - 100	4 - 6	15 - 20	-	
Midazolam (Versed) 1986	96 - 97	2	water soluble; lipid soluble in vivo	IM	5	--	15	0.5 - 1	preop med
				IV	1 - 1.5	--	0.5 - 2	immediate	conscious sedation
				IV	10 - 25	--	0.5 - 2	immediate	anesthesia induction

These benzodiazepines are primarily glucoronidated (excretion rapid; minimal accumulation).

Reprinted with permission from reference 23.

Comparison of Long-Acting Anxiolytics (Benzodiazepines)

Drug and Year of Introduction	Protein Binding (%)	Half-Life (hr)	Solubility	Route	Dose (mg)	Frequency (hr)	Onset (min)	Peak (hr)	Use
Chlordiazepoxide (Librium) 1960	96.5	7 - 28	water soluble	PO	50 - 100	6	15 - 45	0.5 - 2	anxiolytic
			less fat soluble	IM	25 - 100	2 - 4	15 - 30	erratic	
				IV	25 - 100	PRN	1 - 5	immediate	
Clorazepate (Tranxene) 1972	96 - 97	very rapidly metabolized to active metabolites	lipid soluble	PO	7.5 - 30	6 - 8	30 - 60	1 - 2	anxiolytic
Diazepam (Valium) 1963	98.7	20 - 90	insoluble in water; good lipid solubility; distributed in body fat	PO	2 - 10	6	15 - 45	0.5 - 1.5	anxiolytic; sedative; hypnotic; induction agent; anticonvulsant
				IM	2 - 10	3 - 4	20	0.5 - 1.5	
				IV	2 - 10	PRN	1 - 3	immediate	
Flunitrazepam (Rohypnol) 1973	77 - 79	15 - 30	lipid soluble	PO	2	24	30 - 60	1.0 - 1.5	sedative; hypnotic

Drug and Year of Introduction	Protein Binding (%)	Half-Life (hr)	Solubility	Route	Dose (mg)	Frequency (hr)	Onset (min)	Peak (hr)	Use
Flurazepam (Dalmane)	88	very rapidly metabolized; active metabolites last 24 - 100 hr	water soluble	PO	15 - 30	24	15 - 45	0.5 - 1	sedative-hypnotic
Halazepam (Paxipam) 1981	very high	14	lipid soluble	PO	20 - 40	6 - 8	varies	1 - 3	anxiolytic
Nitrazepam (Mogadon) 1964	87	18 - 34	lipid soluble	PO	5	24	15 - 45	1.5	sedative-hypnotic
Prazepam (Centrax)	85 - 90	63 - 70	lipid soluble	PO	5 - 40	8	240 - 360	6 (peak of major metabolite)	anxiolytic

Primarily dealkylated, then usually slowly glucoronidated; accumulation occurs with repeated doses.

Reprinted with permission from reference 23.

Comparison of Nonbarbiturate Sedative-Hypnotics

Drug	Protein Binding (%)	Half-Life (hr)	Route	Sedative Dose (mg)	Hypnotic Dose (mg)	Onset (min)	Duration (hr)	Metab/Excr	Comments
Chloral hydrate (Noctec) and its metabolite	--	--	PO PR	250 325	500 - 1000 500 - 1000	30 30	4 - 8 4 - 8	Met - in RBCs and liver to active metabolite - trichloroethanol; also in liver and kidney to inactive metabolites Excr - renal and bile	give after meals or with glass of fluid to reduce gastric irritation
Trichloro-ethanol	70 - 80	7 - 10							
Ethchlorvynol (Placidyl)	35 - 50	10 - 20	PO	NU	500 - 1000	15 - 60	5	Met - 90% hepatic slight renal Excr - renal	give with food or drink; delirium with TCAs; avoid with porphyria
Ethinamate (Valmid)	--	5 - 33	PO	NU	500 - 1000	20 - 30	3 - 5	Met - hepatic Excr - renal	no hangover or gastric irritation; paradoxical excitement in children
Glutethimide (Doriden)	50	10 - 12	PO	NU	250 - 500	30	4 - 8	Met - hepatic Excr - renal, 2% fecal	may cause leukopenia or thrombocytopenic purpura

Drug	Protein Binding (%)	Half-Life (hr)	Route	Sedative Dose (mg)	Hypnotic Dose (mg)	Onset (min)	Duration (hr)	Metab/Excr	Comments
Meprobamate (Equanil, Miltown)	--	10	PO	NU	400	20 - 40	6 - 8	Met - hepatic Excr - renal	may cause thrombocytopenic purpura
Methyprylon (Noludar)	60	3 - 6	PO	NU	200 - 400	45	5 - 8	Met - hepatic Excr - renal	dependency rare
Paraldehyde (Paral)	--	3.5 9.5	PO PR IM IV	5 - 10 ml 5 - 10 ml 2 - 5 ml 5 ml (dilute)	10 - 30 ml 10 - 30 ml 10 ml 10 ml (dilute)	15 15 15 rapid	8 8 8 8	Met - 80% hepatic Excr - 80% renal 20% pulmonary	characteristic odor on breath; discard if brown; use glass syringe

NU = not used.

These drugs are subject to abuse and are in Schedule IV. Slow withdrawal recommended to avoid convulsions and other symptoms.

Reprinted with permission from reference 24.

Comparison of Benzodiazepines, Phenothiazines, and Butyrophenones

System or Organ	Benzodiazepines	Phenothiazines	Butyrophenones
Central nervous			
General	hypnotic-sedatives; reduce aggression; not cataleptics; cause amnesia	stimulate reticular system; decrease responsiveness; cataleptics; cause amnesia	sedative; cause indifference to stimuli; do not produce sleep; cataleptic and taming effect; impair conditioned reflexes and learning
Hypothalamus	do not affect control of temperature	depress and impair control of temperature	reduce mortality from stress and trauma; lower temperature
Limbic system	anticonvulsants	toxic dose cause amygdalic seizures	toxic dose cause amygdalic seizures
Basal ganglia	no tonic, clonic, or extra-pyramidal effects	lower tone; cause extra-pyramidal dyskinesia and parkinsonism	lower tone; causes extra-pyramidal dyskinesia and and parkinsonism
Chemoreceptor trigger zone	no clinical effect	protect against apo-morphine induced emesis	droperidol long-acting anti-emetic; lowers CSF pressure
Peripheral nerves	no effect	no effect	local anesthetic effect
Autonomic nerves	no effect	alpha-adrenergic and muscarinic blockade	alpha-adrenergic and dopaminergic blockade

System or Organ	Benzodiazepines	Phenothiazines	Butyrophenones
Muscles	multisynaptic central muscle relaxation	mild relaxant of spastic muscles	no clinically useful muscle relaxation
Endocrine	no increase of prolactin and milk production	hypothalamic infertility; lactation and testicular atrophy	like phenothiazines, increased prolactin may cause galactorrhea
Kidney	enuresis; failure of ejaculation occurs rarely	diuretic action; lower antidiuretic output	diuretic action; lower antidiuretic output
Cardiovascular	vasodilation and bradycardia only in large doses	hypotension "central and peripheral effect"; cardiac depressant; negative inotropic effect	protects against catecholamines; lower blood pressure and pulse; no depressant effect on heart
Toxicity	skin rash; nausea; headache; impaired sexual function; vertigo; irregular menses	increased bile viscosity; cholestatic jaundice; skin reactions; parkinsonism; hypotension; blood dyscrasias (rarely); neuroleptic malignant syndrome	increased plasma glutamic pyruvic transaminase; leukopenia and agranulocytosis neuroleptic malignant syndrome
Uses	anxiolytic-sedative; hypnotic; anesthesia adjunct	antipsychotic; antiparkinsonism; antihistaminic; antiemetic	antipsychotic; chronic pain; controls coprolalia and tic in Gilles de la Tourette's Syndrome; neuroleptic anesthesia

Reprinted with permission from reference 23.

Comparison of Barbiturates

Drug	Protein Binding (%)	Half-Life (hr)	pKa	Renal Excretion (% Unchanged)	Sedative Dose (mg), Frequency	Hypnotic Dose (mg)	Comments
Ultrashort Acting (given IV, duration 5 - 20 min[a])							
Methohexital (Brevital)	--	--	8.05	--	used for IV induction 0.5 - 1.5 mg/kg	--	some muscular twitching
Thiamylal (Surital)	--	--	--	--	used for IV induction 1 - 2 mg/kg	--	
Thiopental (Pentothal)	80	3 - 8	7.4	0.3	used for IV induction 1 - 5 mg/kg	--	rare bronchospasm; 99.7% metabolized in liver
Short Acting (onset orally 10 - 15 min, duration 3 - 4 hr)							
Hexobarbital (Sombulex)	42 - 52	2.7 - 7	8.34	--	not used	250 - 500	high abuse potential
Pentobarbital (Nembutal)	60 - 70	15 - 48	8.0	1	30 6 - 12 hr	90 - 180	may be given PO, PR, IV or IM high abuse potential
Secobarbital (Seconal)	46 - 70	19 - 34	7.9	5	30 - 50 6 - 8 hr	100	may be given PO, PR, IV or IM high abuse potential

Drug	Protein Binding (%)	Half-Life (hr)	pKa	Renal Excretion (% Unchanged)	Sedative Dose (mg), Frequency	Hypnotic Dose (mg)	Comments
Intermediate Acting (onset oral 45 - 60 min, duration 6 - 8 hr)							
Amobarbital (Amytal)	61	8 - 42	7.93	1	22 - 50 8 - 12 hr	100 - 200	high abuse potential
Aprobarbital (Alurate)	--	14 - 34	8.09	13 - 24	40 - 80 8 hr	40 - 160	--
Butabarbital (Butisol)	26	34 - 42	--	1	7.5 - 60 6 - 8 hr	100 - 200	--
Talbutal (Lotusate)	--	--	--	trace	30 8 - 12 hr	120	--
Long Acting (onset oral 60 min or more, duration 10 -12 hr)							
Metharbital (Gemonil)	--	--	8.3	2	used as anticonvulsant 100 - 200 mg / 8 hr		--
Mephobarbital (Mebaral)	40 - 60	--	11 - 67	25	32 - 100 6 - 8 hr	not used	--
Phenobarbital (Luminal)	20 - 45	24 - 140	7.3	25	15 - 30 8 - 12 hr	100 - 200	may be given PO, IM, or IV; significant hepatic enzyme induction

[a]Short duration due to redistribution, long duration due to hepatic metabolism.

Reprinted with permission from reference 24.

Agents Used in Premedication and Intraoperative Sedation in Children

Drug	Dose (mg/kg)	Route	Onset Time (min)	Advantages/DisaclvantaRes
Ketamine	1 - 2	IV	<5	Rapid onset, reliable; secretions ↑ (give atropine), may cause apnea (IV), blunts airway responses, sterile abscess (IM)
Fentanyl	0.001 - 0.005	IV	<5	Rapid, reliable; IV route threatening and painful
Midazolam	0.01 - 0.03	IV	<5	Reliable sedation; unpleasant taste (IN and PO) (PO mix with syrup), absorption can be delayed (PR)
	0.05 - 0.1	IM	5 - 10	
	0.1 - 0.2	IN	15 - 30	
	0.5 - 0.6	PO	15 - 30	
	1 - 3	PR	10	
Methohexital	25 - 30	PR	5 - 10	± painful; onset unreliable, hiccups
Chloral hydrate	30 - 100	PO, PR	30 - 60	Sedation, unpleasant taste, slow onset

IV, intravenous; IM, intramuscular; PO, oral; PR, rectal; IN, intranasal.

Modified with permission from reference 25.

Pharmacology

Neuromuscular Blocking Agents and Related Drugs

Comparison of Nondepolarizing and Depolarizing Neuromuscular Blocking Agents

	Nondepolarizing	Depolarizing
Produces fasciculations	no	yes
Fade with repeated stimulation	yes	no
Posttetanic potentiation	yes	no
Effect of Anticholinesterase	reversal	potentiation
Effect antagonized by	depolarizing agents	nondepolarizing agents

Tests for Neuromuscular Transmission

Test	Percent of Receptors Occupied	Disadvantages
Tidal volume	80	Insensitive
Sustained tetanus at 30 Hz	75 - 80	Insensitive & uncomfortable
Twitch height	75 - 80	Insensitive, uncomfortable, and requires knowledge of patient's twitch prior to administration of neuromuscular blocker
Vital capacity	70 - 75	Insensitive and requires patient cooperation
Train-of-four	70 - 75	Not very sensitive
Sustained tetanus at 100 Hz	50	Very painful
Inspiratory force	50	Difficult to perform when patient is not intubated
Head lift and hand grip	33	Need cooperation of patient

Muscle Relaxants

Drug	Onset (min)	Duration (min)	Spontaneous Recovery (min)	Priming Dose (mg/kg)	ED95 (mg/kg)	Intubation Dose (mg/kg)
Ultra-Short						
Succinylcholine	1	5 - 10	20	-	0.50	1 - 2
Short						
Mivacurium	2 - 2.5	15 - 20	25 - 30	0.02 - 0.03	0.07	0.15
Rocuronium	1 - 1.5	20 - 35	30 - 50	0.1	0.3	0.6
Intermediate						
Atracurium	3 - 5	20 - 35	40 - 60	0.05 - 0.06	0.232	0.4 - 0.5
Vecuronium	3 - 5	20 - 35	40 - 60	0.01 - 0.015	0.05	0.08 - 0.1
Cisatracurium	1.5 - 2*	40 - 60	60 - 80	0.02	0.05	0.2*
Long†						
d-Tubocurarine	4 - 6	45 - 60	60 - 180	0.04 - 0.05	0.51	0.5 - 0.6
Metocurine	4 - 6	45 - 60	60 - 180	0.02 - 0.03	0.28	0.3 - 0.4
Pancuronium	4 - 6	45 - 60	60 - 180	0.01 - 0.15	0.07	0.1
Doxacurium	4 - 6	45 - 60	60 - 180	0.005	0.025	0.05 - 0.08‡
Pipecuronium	4 - 6	45 - 60	60 - 180	0.01 - 0.02	0.07	0.1

* = for children 2 - 12 yrs, faster onset and shorter duration; use 0.1 mg/kg for intubation dose;
† = large individual variability; ‡ = use larger dose (i.e., 0.08 mg/kg) only for longer cases.

Muscle Relaxants

Drug	Maintenance N_2O/Opioid (mg/kg)	Maintenance Volatile Agent (mg/kg)	Maintenance N_2O/Opioid Infusion Rate (mg/kg/min)	Maintenance Volatile Agent Infusion Rate (mg/kg/min)	Comments
Ultra-Short					
Succinylcholine	-	-	50 - 100	30 - 50	Shortest onset and duration; plasma cholinesterase-dependent; side effects include hyperkalemia, possible bradycardia
Short					
Mivacurium	0.1	0.075	6 - 7	4 - 6	Plasma cholinesterase-dependent
Rocuronium	0.15	0.1	8 - 9	5 - 6	Shortest onset for nondepolarizing drug
Intermediate					
Atracurium	0.1	0.05	5 - 9	3 - 6	Lacks hepatic and renal metabolism; histamine release with larger doses
Vecuronium	0.02	0.01	1 - 2	0.6 - 1.2	Minimal cardiovascular effects; some bradycardia observed; no histamine release observed
Cisatracurium	0.03	0.02	2 - 3	1 - 2	No histamine release with usual doses
Long					
d-Tubocurarine	0.1	0.05	-	-	Ganglion blocker; histamine release observed
Metocurine	0.07	0.04	-	-	Fewer side effects compared to d-Tubocurarine
Pancuronium	0.015	0.005	1 - 2	0.6 - 1.2	Cardiovascular side effects; vagolytic action
Doxacurium	0.025	0.01	-	-	Minimal cardiovascular side effects
Pipecuronium	0.01	0.005	-	-	Minimal cardiovascular side effects

Anticholinesterase Agents

	Dosage (mg/kg)	Peak Antagonism (min)	Duration Of Antagonism (min)	Dosage Of Atropine (μg/kg)	Dosage Of Glyco-pyrrolate (μg/kg)	Metabolism and Comments
Edrophonium (Tensilon)	0.5 - 1.0	1 - 3	45 - 60	7 - 10	10	30% hepatic; duration prolonged in renal failure; may cause bradycardia, hypotension, CNS stimulation or depression, GI cramps or cholinergic crisis; due to the difference in onset times, administer glycopyrrolate several minutes in advance
Neostigmine (Prostigmin)	0.03 - 0.07 (up to 5 mg)	7 - 10	55 - 75	15 - 30	10 - 15	50% hepatic; duration prolonged in renal failure; may cause bradycardia, hypotension, CNS stimulation or depression, GI cramps or cholinergic crisis.
Pyridostigmine (Regonol; Mestinon)	0.25	10 - 13	80 - 130	15 - 20	10	75% hepatic; duration prolonged in renal failure; does not significantly cross the blood-brain barrier; not recommended for use with atropine due to the differences in onset times; therapy for myasthenia gravis

Anticholinergic Agents*

Drug	Onset (min)	Duration (min)	Effect On Heart Rate	Effect On CNS	Effect On Secretions	Effect On Smooth Muscle Tone
Atropine	1 - 1.5	15 - 30	↑↑↑	Mild Sedation	↓↓	↓↓
Glycopyrrolate	4 - 5	120 - 240	↑↑	None	↓↓↓	↓↓↓

*Used principally to antagonize the muscarinic effects of anticholinesterase agents (e.g., edrophonium and neostigmine). Additional uses include bronchial dilation in patients with reactive airway disease.

See previous page for dose range for a given anticholinesterase agent.

Pharmacology

Intravenous Anesthetic Agents

Properties of Intravenous Anesthetic Drugs (part 1)

Drug and Date of Introduction	Mol Wt	pK_a	Solution pH	Induction Dose (mg/kg)	Half-life	Volume of Distribution (L/kg)	Clearance (mL/kg/min)
Amobarbital (Amytal) 1930	248.26	7.94	9.6	2 - 4	alpha - short beta 14 - 42 hr	0.9 - 1.4	0.5 - 0.6
Thiopental (Pentothal) 1934	264.32	7.45	10.5 - 11	4 - 5	alpha 10 - 14 min beta 3 - 8 hr	2.5 ± 1	3.4 ± 0.5
Thiamylal (Surital) 1950	276.33	7.48	10.5 - 11	4 - 5	alpha 8 - 12 min	N/A	N/A
Methohexital (Brevital) 1957	284.30	7.9	10 - 11	1 - 1.5	alpha 4 - 6 min beta 1.5 - 4 hr	2.1 ± 0.7	9.9 ± 2.9
Propanidid (Epontal) 1961	337.4	N/A	5.4 - 6.0	5 - 10	alpha 3 min beta 0.2 hr	0.5	34 - 35
Diazepam (Valium) 1966 (IV)	284.74	3.4	6.2 - 6.9	0.5	pi 2 - 13 min alpha 1 -3 hr beta 12 - 37 hr	1.86	0.38
Droperidol (Inaspine)1963	379.42	7.64	3.4	0.25	alpha 10 min beta 134 ± 13 min	2.54	16 - 17
Ketamine (Ketalar) 1970	274.19	7.5	3.5 - 5.5	1 - 2 IV 2 - 10 IM	alpha 10 - 15 min beta 2.5 hr	1 - 3	17

Drug and Date of Introduction	Mol Wt	pK_a	Induction Solution pH	Dose (mg/kg)	Half-life	Volume of Distribution (L/kg)	Clearance (mL/kg/min)
Alphaxalone-alphadolone (Althesin) 1972	alphax 33.249 alphad 390.62	N/A	7.0	0.05 - 0.1 mg/kg	alpha 2.4 min beta 34 min	0.79	18 - 19
Etomidate (Amidate) 1972	244.29	4.24	4 - 7	0.2 - 0.4	pi 2.6 ± 1.3 min alpha 28.7 min beta 4.6 ± 2.6 hr	4.6	13 - 15
Lorazepam (Ativan) 1980	321.16	1.3 and 11.5	6.4	0.1 - 0.15	alpha 8.7 ± 1.9 min beta 16 hr	1.32	1.2
Midazolam (Versed) 1986	362.23	6.2	3.5	0.2	alpha 5 - 8 min beta 1.7 - 2.0 hr	1.72	6 - 8
Propofol (Diprivan)	178.27	11.1	6.0 - 8.5	2.5	alpha 1.8 - 8.3 min beta 34 - 64 min	5 - 20	20 - 30

Modified with permission from reference 26.

Properties of Intravenous Anesthetic Drugs (part 2)

	Protein LD_{50} (mg/kg)	ED_{50} (mg/kg)	Binding (%)	Lipid Solubility	Water Solubility	Metabolism and Metabolite	Route of Elimination
Amobarbital	rat 115 IP	N/A	61	high	soluble	liver	renal
Thiopental	mouse 78 IV	2.63	75 - 80	high	soluble	liver rate 16-24%/hr thiopental-carboxylic acid	renal
Thiamylal	N/A	N/A	high	high	soluble	liver	renal
Methohexital	rat 33.2	1.1	73	high	soluble	liver by hydroxylation	fecal
Propanidid	cat 80 - 90	3.66	40	high	moderate to low	pseudocholinesterase and hepatic hydrolysis	90% renal 6% fecal
Diazepam	mouse 500 - 950 oral	0.5 IV	98	high	low to insoluble	liver, desmethyldiazepam (90% as active) hydroxydiazepam	70% renal 10% fecal
Droperidol	rabbit 97 mouse 200	N/A	85 - 90	high	moderate	liver	75% renal 22% fecal
Ketamine	rat 224 IP	N/A	human low cat 50	high	soluble	liver demethylation and hydroxylation, norketamine (one-third as active)	91% renal 3% fecal

	Protein LD$_{50}$ (mg/kg)	ED$_{50}$ (mg/kg)	Binding (%)	Lipid Solubility	Water Solubility	Metabolism and Metabolite	Route of Elimination
Alphaxalone-alphadolone	54.7	0.14	35 - 50	low	low	liver hydroxylation and conjugation	56% renal
Etomidate	15.1	rat 0.57	76.5	high	soluble but unstable	liver by hydrolysis	77.8% renal 12.9% fecal
Lorazepam	24 - 50 IV	0.07 oral	93	mod-erate	insoluble	liver by conjugation to lorazepam glucuronide	88% renal 7% fecal
Midazolam	450 oral	0.15 IV	95	high	soluble	liver by conjugation to 4-hydroxy- and 1-hydroxymethyl-	renal
Propofol	rat 42 IV	mouse 12.8	98	high	low	liver by conjugation to glucuronide	renal

Modified with permission from reference 26.

Pharmacology

Cardiovascular Drugs

Properties of Adrenergic Agonists

Drug	Intestinal Absorption	Route	Dose (mg)	Peak Effect	Frequency (hr)	Metabolism	Excretion	Comments
Active at alpha and beta receptors								
Norepinephrine (Levophed)	poor	IV	2 - 4 μg/min	3 - 10 min	infusion	COMT[a] MAO[b]	renal	catecholamine[c]; levarterenol vasoconstrictor; noradrenaline poorly absorbed IM, SC
Epinephrine Adrenaline (Adrenalin)	poor	inhalation	0.16	-	-	COMT MAO	renal	catecholamine; vasoconstrictor; poorly absorbed IM, SC (vasodilates IM)
		SC	0.1 - 0.5	-	4			
		IV	0.1 - 0.25	3 - 10 min	infusion			
		topical/ rectal	0.25% - 2%	-	—			
Dopamine (Intropin)	-	IV	1 - 10 μg/ kg/min	2 - 10 min	infusion	COMT MAO	renal	catecholamine; renal vasodilator
Ephedrine	interme- diate	oral	25 - 50	0.5 - 2 hr	3 - 4 repeat if necessary	hepatic	renal	direct and indirect acting
		IV	5 - 25	-				
		IM	12.5 - 50	-				
		SC	12.5 - 50	-				
Amphetamine (Benzedrine)	rapid	oral	5 - 20	30 - 60 min	8 - 24	hepatic	renal	excretion increased in acidic urine; direct and indirect acting
Selective for alpha 1-receptor (vasoconstriction)								
Phenylephrine (Neosynephrine)	-	topical	0.125 - 1%	2 - 5 min	4 - 6	hepatic intestinal	renal	vasoconstrictor; poorly absorbed IM, SC
		IV	0.2	immediate	10 -15 min			
		IM	2 - 5	15-30 min	10 -15 min			
		SC	2 - 5	15-30 min	10 -15 min			

Drug	Intestinal Absorption	Route	Dose (mg)	Peak Effect	Frequency (hr)	Metabolism	Excretion	Comments
Metaraminol (Aramine)	-	IV SC IM	0.5 - 5 2 - 10 2 - 10	2 - 5 min 10 - 20 min 10 - 20 min	Then infusion as needed	hepatic	renal biliary	light sensitive, vasoconstrictor; poorly absorbed IM, SC; precipitates acidic drugs
Methoxamine (Vasoxyl)	-	IV IM	3 - 10 slow 10 - 15	immediate 15 - 30 min	15 -30 min if needed	-	-	vasoconstrictor;poorly absorbed IM, SC
Selective for alpha 2-receptors (antihypertensives)								
Clonidine (Catapres)	good	oral	0.1 - 0 2	3 - 5 hr	6 - 12	hepatic	renal 65%, biliary 20%	
Methyldopa (Aldomet)	about 50%	oral IV	250 - 500 250 - 500	4 -6 hr infuse over	6 - 12 6 hr	neuron; liver/conjugation	renal, fecal	metabolized to active product, methyl norepinephrine
Guanabenz (Wytensin)	75% 16%	oral	4 - 16	2 - 4 hr	12	hepatic	renal, fecal	extensive first pass metabolism
Active at beta 1- and beta 2-receptor (bronchodilator and cardiotonic)								
Isoproterenol Isoprenaline (Isuprel)	erratic	inhalation IV IM SC oral	0.12 - 0.24 0.01 - 0.02 0.2 - 1.0 0.15 - 0.2 5 - 15	0.25 - 1 min 3 - 10 min 10-20 min 10-20 min 10 - 30 min	4 - 6 as needed as needed as needed 6 - 8	liver, lungs COMT MAO	renal	catecholamine vasodilator; well absorbed parenterally
Selective for beta 1-receptor (cardiotonic)								
Dobutamine (Dobutrex)	-	IV	2.5 - 10 µg/kg/min	2 - 10 min	infusion	hepatic	renal	catecholamine

Properties of Adrenergic Agonists (continued)

Drug	Intestinal Absorption	Route	Dose (mg)	Peak Effect	Frequency (hr)	Metabolism	Excretion	Comments
Selective for beta 2-receptors (bronchodilator or tocolytic)								
Isoetharine (Bronkosol)	-	inhalation	1.5	15 - 60 min	4	lungs, liver, intestines	renal	aerosol; rapidly absorbed
Metaproterenol (Alupent)	40%	inhalation	1.3 - 1.95	60 min	6 - 8	hepatic	renal	light-sensitive; aerosol absorbed slowly
		oral	10 - 20	60 min	6 - 8			
Terbutaline (Brethine)	slow	oral	5	2 - 3 hr	6	hepatic	renal	light sensitive
		SC	0.25 - 0.5	30 - 60 min	4			
		IV	10 - 80	30 - 60 min	infusion			
Albuterol	well	inhalation	0.18	60 - 90 min	4 - 6	hepatic	renal,	light-sensitive; aerosol
Salbutamol (Proventil, Ventolin)		oral	2 - 4	6 hr	6 - 8		fecal 4 - 10%	absorbed slowly
Ritodrine (Yutopar)	30%	oral	10	10 - 60 min	2	hepatic	renal	tocolytic; for premature labor; avoid in diabetics; may cause hypokalemia and pulmonary edema
		IV	50 - 350 µg/min	5 - 60 min	infusion			

[a]COMT = catechol-O-methyltransferase; [b]MAO = monoamine oxidase
[c]Catecholamines are readily oxidized; do not mix with alkaline solutions; ineffective orally

Modified with permission from reference 27.

Properties of Adrenergic Antagonists

Drug	Intestinal Absorption	Route	Dose (mg)	Peak Effect	Frequency (hr)	Metabolism	Excretion	Comments
Block alpha 1- and alpha 2-receptors (for pheochromocytoma, malignant hypertension)								
Phentolamine (Regitine)	-	IV	2.5 - 5	1 - 5 min	as needed	hepatic	renal	for diagnosis of pheochromocytoma
Phenoxybenzemine (Dibenzyline)	variable	oral	10 - 20	1 - 2 days	8	hepatic	renal, biliary	
Selective blockade at alpha 1-receptors (for hypertension)								
Prazosin (Minipress)	good	oral	0.5 - 5	2 - 4 hr	8 - 12	hepatic	biliary, renal 10%	
Block beta 1- and beta 2-receptors (for angina, arrhythmias, and hypertension)								
Propranolol (Inderal)	good	oral IV	10 - 80 1 - 3	1 - 1.5 hr 1 - 2 min	8 - 12 2 min, then 4 hr	hepatic	renal 90%, 1% unchanged	first-pass effect; 90% bound to plasma protein membrane stabilizer
Timolol (Blocadren)	variable	oral	10 - 30	1 - 2 hr	12	hepatic	renal 60%, 20% unchanged	
Nadolol (Corgard)	variable	oral	40 - 320	4 hr	24	hepatic	renal 90%, 40% unchanged	
Pindolol (Visken)	variable	oral	5 - 30	1 - 2 hr	24	hepatic	renal 90%, 40% unchanged	partial agonist; membrane stabilizer

Drug	Intestinal Absorption	Route	Dose (mg)	Peak Effect	Frequency (hr)	Metabolism	Excretion	Comments
Selective blockade at beta 1-receptors (for angina and hypertension)								
Atenolol (Tenormin)	-	oral	50 - 100	2 - 4 hr	24	none	renal, 40% unchanged	
Metoprolol (Lopressor)	variable	oral	100 - 450	1 - 2 hr	24	hepatic	renal 90% 3% unchanged	
Block alpha 1- and beta 1-receptors (for hypertension)								
Labetalol (Trandate)	good	oral	100 - 400	2 - 3 hr	12	hepatic	renal 60%, 5% unchanged	alpha blockade at higher doses

Reprinted with permission from reference 27.

Drugs Used in the Management of Pheochromocytoma

Drug	Action	Route	Dose	Route	Dose	Comments
Phentolamine	α-blocker	IV	2 - 5 mg	--	--	Rapid onset, short-acting; give bolus every 5 min or initially 1 mg/min
Phenoxy-benzamine	α-blocker	--	--	PO	30 mg/day increasing daily dosage by 30 mg	Long half-life; may accumulate; give 2 - 3 times daily
Prazosin	α-blocker	--	--	PO	1.0 mg single dose, increasing to TID	May cause syncope, so start with low dose before bedtime; first dose phenomenon regimen
Propranolol	β-blocker	IV	1.0 mg bolus to total of 10 mg	PO	40 mg BID; increase to 480 mg/day	When used alone may cause syncope, so start with low dose
Atenolol	β-blocker	--	--	PO	50 mg/day initially; may increase to 100 mg/day	Long-acting selective β_1 antagonist eliminated by kidney
Esmolol	β-blocker	IV	500 μg/kg/min loading followed by maintenance infusion	--	--	Ultra short-acting selective β_1 antagonist may be used during anesthesia
Labetalol	α-and β-blocker	IV	10 mg bolus to 150 mg	PO	200 mg TID	A much weaker α-blocker than β-blocker; may cause pressor response in pheochromocytoma; powerful vasodilator short-acting; may be used during anesthesia

Drug	Action	Route	Dose	Route	Dose	Comments
Nitroprusside	Vasodilator	IV	Infusion initially 0.5 - 1.5 μg/kg/min	--	--	Powerful vasodilator; short-acting; may be used during anesthesia
α-Methyl-tyrosine	Inhibition of catecholamine biosynthesis	--	--	PO	1 - 4 gm/day	Suitable for patients not amenable to surgery; may be nephrotoxic

Reproduced with permission from reference 28.

Pharmacologic Characteristics Antihypertensive Drugs for Oral Administration to Pediatric Patients

Drug	Administration: Preparation	Administration: Dosage	Interval for Dose Increase	Removal by Dialysis: H	Removal by Dialysis: P	Adverse Effects	Relative Contraindications	Comments
β-Adrenergic Blocking Drugs								
Propranolol (Inderal)	Tablets: 10,20, 40, 50 mg	0.5 - 1 mg/kg/d ÷ Q 6 h	3 - 6 d	-	-	Cardiovascular: bradycardia, congestive heart failure, intensification of AV block CNS: mental depression (insomnia, lassitude, weakness, fatigue), visual disturbances, disorientation, emotional liability, hallucinations, nightmares) Respiratory: bronchospasm Gastrointestinal: nausea, vomiting, diarrhea	Asthma Congestive heart failure Sinus bradycardia, Heart block greater than 1° Diabetes Active liver disease Pheochromocytoma (before α-blockade) Cardiogenic shock	Inhibits reflex tachycardia (exercise, posture vasodilators) May mask signs of hyperthyroidism and hypoglycemia Action potentiated by diuretics

Drug	Administration		Interval for Dose	Removal by Dialysis			Relative	
	Preparation	Dosage	Increase	H	P	Adverse Effects	Contraindications	Comments
Atenolol† (Tenormin)	Tablets: 50, 100 mg	50 mg Q d (adult dose)	7 - 14 d	+	-	Has the fewest side effects	Can be used cautiously in asthmatics	Relatively cardioselective
Metoprolol† (Lopressor)	Tablets: 50, 100 mg	1 mg/kg Q 12 h*	7 d			Same as β-blockers but less severe	Same as β-blockers but can be used in asthmatics	Same as β-blockers β_1 selectivity enhanced at low doses β-blocker of choice in asthmatics
Nadolol† (Corgard)	Tablets: 40, 80, 120,160 mg	1 mg/kg Q 24 h*	3 - 7 d	+		Same as β-blockers less severe, especially CNS	Same as β-blockers	Same as β-blockers Longer duration allows once-a-day dosage
Vasodilator Drugs								
Hydralazine (Apresoline)	Tablets: 10, 25 50, 100 mg (unstable in solution)	0.75 - 3 mg/kg/d ÷ Q 4 - 6 h to a max. of 200 mg Q 24 h	3 - 4 d	-	-	Vasodilation symptoms sweating, flushing feelings of warmth, orthostatic hypotension tachycardia palpitations, nausea, and vomiting	Tachycardia Hypersensitivity to hydralazine	Unstable in suspension Periodic LE prep and and ANA should be done

Pharmacologic Characteristics Antihypertensive Drugs for Oral Administration to Pediatric Patients (cont.)

Drug	Administration Preparation	Administration Dosage	Interval for Dose Increase	Removal by Dialysis H	Removal by Dialysis P	Adverse Effects	Relative Contraindications	Comments
Minoxidil (Loniten)	Tablets: 2.5, 10 mg	0.1 - 0.2 mg/kg Q 8 - 24 h to a max of 50 mg for < 12 y; 100 mg for > 12 y	3 d (can be every 6 h with care)	+	+	Headache Vasodilation symptoms, sweating, flushing feelings of warmth, orthostatic hypotension tachycardia, palpitations, nausea, and vomiting Hypertrichosis Sodium retention Ascites Pericardial effusion	Pheochromocytoma	Always use with a diuretic May cause severe hypotension in patients on guanethidine Discontinue gradually
Angiotensin Converting Enzyme Inhibitor Drugs								
Captopril (Capoten)	Tablets: 25, 50, 100 mg (unstable in suspension)	0.15 mg/kg (Infants: 0.05 - 0.1 mg/kg)	Dose to dose	+		Rash Hyperkalemia (patients with renal failure) Proteinuria Neutropenia	Renal artery stenosis Volume contraction	Presence of food decreases absorption by 30 - 40%; give a.c. Action potentiated by diuretics Causes false-positive urine acetone

Drug	Administration: Preparation	Administration: Dosage	Interval for Dose Increase	Removal by Dialysis: H	Removal by Dialysis: P	Adverse Effects	Relative Contraindications	Comments
Enalapril¥ (Vasotec)	Tablets: 2.5, 5, 10, 20 mg	2.5 - 5 mg Q d (adult dose); twice a day for more even control	2 - 3 d (takes weeks for full effect)	+		Same as captopril	Same as captopril	Absorption unaffected by food
Calcium Channel-Blocking Drugs								
Nifedipine (Procardia)	Capsules: 10, 20 mg	0.25 mg/kg Q 4 - 6 h	Dose to dose			Vasodilation Tachycardia Sweating Nausea Vomiting	Concomitant use of β-blocking drugs or cimetidine	Absorption unaffected by food
Nifedipine extended release (Nifedipine)	Tablets: 30, 60 mg	30 mg Q d (adult dose)	7 - 14 d			Same as nifedipine	Same as nifedipine	Same as nifedipine
Verapamil (Calan)	Tablets: 40, 80, 120 mg	4 - 10 mg/kg/d ÷ 3 times a day	5-7 d			Same as nifedipine	Same as nifedipine	Absorption delayed by food

Pharmacologic Characteristics Antihypertensive Drugs for Oral Administration to Pediatric Patients (cont.)

Drug	Administration Preparation	Administration Dosage	Interval for Dose Increase	Removal by Dialysis H	Removal by Dialysis P	Adverse Effects	Relative Contraindications	Comments
Central Adrenergic Stimulating Drugs								
Clonidine** (Catapres)	Tablets: 0.1, 0.2, 0.3 mg	0.05 mg/kg twice a day to a max of 2.4 mg Q 24 h	1 - 4 d	-		Dry mouth Sedation/fatigue Retinal degeneration		Action potentiated by diuretics Rebound hypertension if D/C suddenly
α-Adrenergic Blocking Drugs								
Prazosin** (Minipress)	Capsules: 1, 2, 5 mg	1 mg to a max of 20 mg Q 24 h*	2 - 3 d			Orthostatic hypotension Lethargy Sedation/fatigue	Patients already on minoxidil	Action potentiated by diuretics and minoxidil
Phenoxy-benzamine (Dibenzyline)	Capsules: 10 mg (unstable in suspension)¥	0.2 mg/kg Q 24 h	4 d			Nasal congestion Orthostatic hypotension		Specific for catecholamine excess

*Dose frequency may be decreased to bid after BP is controlled. †Manufacturer's warning: Safety and effectiveness in children have not been established. **Manufacturer's warning: No clinical experience for use in children. ¥Instability of this drug in suspension can be circumvented by dissolving tablets/capsules in a measured amount of water and administering immediately.
Abbreviations: H = hemodialysis: P = peritoneal dialysis; + = removed by dialysis,- = not removed by dialysis; AV = atrioventricular; CNS = central nervous system; LE = lupus erythematosus; ANA = antinuclear antibody; a.c. = before meals; D/C = discontinued.

Adapted with permission from reference 29.

Pharmacologic Effects of Antihypertensive Drugs Available for Parenteral and Sublingual Administration to Pediatric Patients

Drug	HR	CO	SVR	RBF*	GFR*
Nitroprusside	V (↑)	V (↓)	↓↓↓	NE	NE
Labetalol	V (↓)	V (↓)	↓	NE	NE
Diazoxide	↑↑	↑	↓↓	↓ then ↑	↓ then V
Hydralazine	↑↑	↑	↓	↑	V (→↓)
Nifedipine	V (↑)	↑	↓↓	NE	NE
Enalaprilat	NE	NE	↓↓	↑↑	↓

*May decrease if patient is dehydrated at time of treatment or if BP is excessively reduced.

Abbreviations: HR = heart rate; CO = cardiac output; SVR = systemic vascular resistance; RBF = renal blood flow; GFR = glomerular filtration rate; NE = no effect; V = variable (arrows in parentheses indicate the more commonly reported effects); ↑/↓ = slightly reduced/increased; ↑↑/↓↓ = moderately reduced/increased; ↓↓↓ = markedly reduced; → = no charge.

Reproduced with permission from reference 29.

Pharmacologic Characteristics Antihypertensive Drugs Available for Parenteral and Sublingual Administration to Pediatric Patients

	Administration			Effect		
Drug	**Route**	**Preparation**	**Dosage**	**Onset**	**Peak**	**Duration**
Sodium nitroprusside**	IV infusion	50 mg of lyophilized powder In D5W	0.5 µg/kg/min titrated to a max of 10 µg/kg/min	Within 30 sec		Length of infusion
Labetalol HCl**	IV bolus injection	20 mL vial containing 100 mg (5 mg/mL)	Bolus: 0.5 mg/kg over 2 min. For nonresponse, double dose and repeat every 10 min to a max dose of 5 mg/kg	1 - 5 min	5 min	Variable
Diazoxide**	IV bolus injection	20 mL ampule containing 300 mg (15 mg/mL)	1 - 3 mg/kg repeated every 5 - 15 min until BP controlled (minibolus)	1 - 5 min	1 - 5 min	Variable Usually less than 12 h
Hydralazine	30 min IV infusion or IM	1 mL ampule containing 20 mg	0.15 - 0.2 mg/kg every 6 hr	10 - 20 min	10 min - 1.5 h	3 - 6 h

		Administration			Effect	
Drug	**Route**	**Preparation**	**Dosage**	**Onset**	**Peak**	**Duration**
Nifedipine	Sublingual	10 and 20 mg capsules	0.25 mg/kg dose 4 - 6 h	10 - 15 min	60 - 90 min	Variable, usually 2 - 4h
Enalaprilat**	IV over 5 min	2 mL vials (1.25 mg/mL)	0.04 - 0.08 mg/kg dose Neonate: 0.01 mg/kg dose	15 min	I - 4 h	Variable
Phentolamine	IV bolus injection	5 mg of lyophilized powder reconstituted with diluent	0.05 - 0.1 mg/kg	Within 30	2 min	15 - 30 min

Adapted with permission from reference 29.

Pharmacologic Characteristics Antihypertensive Drugs Available for Parenteral and Sublingual Administration to Pediatric Patients (continued)

Drug	Removal by Dialysis* H	Removal by Dialysis* P	Adverse Effects	Relative Contraindications	Comments
Sodium nitroprusside	+	+	Nausea/vomiting Vasodilation sx[†] Neurologic sx[¥] Apprehension restlessness	Hepatic insufficiency	Solution good for 24 h Photosensitive (wrap in foil) Monitor blood thiocyanate if used longer than 72 h (D/C for thiocyanate >10 mg/dL)
Labetalol HCl	-	-	Postural hypotension Neurologic sx[†] Nausea/vomiting	Bronchial asthma CHF	Keep supine for 3 h after administering drug Ambulate gradually Use cautiously in pheochromocytoma and diabetes Synergistic with halothane (hypotension)
Diazoxide	+	+	Arrhythmias Hyperglycemia Sodium and water retention Vasodilation sx[†] Neurologic sx[¥]	Thiazide sensitivity Severe tachycardia Diabetes Coarctation	Ineffective in pheochromocytoma Give diuretics to decrease sodium retention Hypoproteinemia potentiates effects Prolonged use (weeks) often reinstates sensitivity to oral medications
Hydralazine	-	-	Headache Nausea/vomiting Tachycardia palpitation	Hypersensitivity to hydralazine ("hyperdynamic syndrome")	Undergoes color change in most infusion fluids, which does not indicate loss of potency

Drug	Removal by Dialysis* H	P	Adverse Effects	Relative Contraindications	Comments
Nifedipine	-	-	Headache Vasodilation sx†	Concomitant use of β-blocking drugs and cimetidine	Dose can be withdrawn from capsule with 1 mL syringe and squirted sublingually
Enalaprilat	+	-	Hypotension when ECFV is contracted Hyperkalemia Oliguria	Renal failure Dehydration	Treat hypotension with volume expansion
Phentolamine			Tachycardia Arrhythmias Marked hypotension		Specific for pheochromocytoma

*Removal of drug for dialysis relates to the need to supplement a dose after dialysis. It does not apply to the use of dialysis to treat drug overdose.

**Manufacturer's warning: safety in children not established.

†Vasodilation symptoms include sweating flushing, feedings of warmth, orthostatic hypotension, tachycardia, palpitations, nausea, and vomiting

¥Neurologic symptoms include headache, blurred vision, dizziness, and lightheadedness.
Abbreviations: sx = symptoms; max = maximum; BP = blood pressure; D5W = 5% dextrose in water; H = hemodialysis; P = peritoneal dialysis; CHF = congestive heart failure; + = removed by dialysis; - = not removed by dialysis; IV = intravenous; D/C = discontinued; HCl = hydrochloride; IM = intramuscular; ECFV = extracellular fluid volume.

Adapted with permission from reference 29.

Pharmacologic Characteristics of Diuretic Drugs for Parenteral and Oral Administration to Pediatric Patients

Drug	Administration		Onset	Peak	Duration
	Preparation	Dosage			
Furosemide (Lasix)	Tablets: 20, 40, 80 mg Oral solution: 10 mg/mL IV: 10 mg/mL	1 - 2 mg increased 1 - 2 mg/kg to a maximum of 6 mg/kg every 24 h	0 - 1 h IV* 5 min IV* 1 h (neonate)	1 - 2 h 30 min 1 - 2 h	4 - 6 h 2 h 5 - 6 h
Ethacrynic acid (Edacrin)	Tablets: 25, 50 mg IV: 50 mg (lyophilized powder reconstituted with D5W)	1 mg/kg increased to 25 mg every 24 hr	0 - 30 min IV: 15 - 30 min	2 h 45 min	6 - 8 h 3 h
Hydrochlorothiazide (HydroDIURIL)	Tablets: 25, 50, 100 mg	2 mg/kg twice daily	2 h	4 h	6 - 12 h
Spironolactone (Aldactone**)	Tablets: 25, 100 mg	1 - 3.3 mg/kg every 6, 8, or 12 h	Gradual	3 d	2 - 3 d

*IV bolus injection should not exceed 4 mg/min to decrease ototoxicity risk.

**Manufacture's warning: Safety and effectiveness in children have not been established.

Abbreviations: IV = intravenous; D5W = dextrose 5% in water.

Pharmacologic Characteristics of Diuretic Drugs for Parenteral and Oral Administration to Pediatric Patients (continued)

Drug	Adverse Effects	Relative Contraindications	Comments
Furosemide	Fluid and electrolyte depletion Hyperuricemia Hyperglycemia	Anuria Metabolic alkalosis Sulfonamide sensitivity	See ethacrynic acid Ototoxicity less than ethacrynic acid
Ethacrynic acid	Fluid and electrolyte depletion Hyperuricemia Hyperglycemia	Anuria Metabolic alkalosis	Periodic determination of serum electrolytes should be performed Ototoxicity with parenteral administration
Hydrochlorothiazide	Electrolyte depletion Hyperuricemia Hyperglycemia	Anuria Sulfonamide sensitivity	Periodic determination of serum electrolytes should be performed Not effective alone, usually use with thiazide (Aldactazide)
Spironolactone	Hyperkalemia Gynecomastia Hyperkalemia	Anuria Rapidly decreasing renal function	

Adapted with permission from reference 29.

Drugs of Choice for Common Arrhythmias

Arrhythmia	Drug of choice	Alternatives	Remarks
Atrial fibrillation or flutter	Verapamil, diltiazem or a beta-blocker to slow ventricular response[1]	Digoxin to slow ventriculi-lar response Quinidine, procainamide, disopyramide, flecainide, propafenone or sotalol for long-term prevention Ibutilide for termination of the arrhythmia	Digoxin, verapamil, diltiazem and possibly beta-blockers may be dangerous for patients with Wolff-Parkinson-White syndrome. Amiodarone in low doses has also been effective for prevention. Radiofrequency catheter ablation has been used in selected patients.
Other supraventricular tachycardias[2]	Adenosine, verapamil[3] or diltiazem[3] for termination	Esmolol, another beta-blocker or digoxin for termination	DC cardioversion or atrial pacing may be effective for some patients. Radiofrequency catheter ablation can cure many patients. Quinidine, procainamide, disopyramide, diltiazem, beta-blockers, verapamil, flecainide, propafenone or digoxin may be effective for long-term suppression.
Ventricular premature complexes (PVCs) or non-sustained ventricular tachycardia	No drug therapy indicated for asymptomatic patients	For symptomatic patients, a beta-blocker	There is no evidence that prolonged suppression with drugs prevents sudden cardiac death. For post-MI patients, treatment with a beta-blocker has decreased mortality, and treatment with flecainide or moricizine has increased it.

Drugs of Choice for Common Arrhythmias

Arrhythmia	Drug of choice	Alternatives	Remarks
Sustained ventricular tachycardia[4,5]	Lidocaine for acute treatment[4,5]	Procainamide, bretylium, amiodarone[4,5]	Sotalol, other beta-blockers, procainamide, quinidine, amiodarone, disopyramide, flecainide, propafenone or mexiletine may be effective for long-term prevention.[6]
Ventricular fibrillation[7]	Lidocaine[7]	Amiodarone, procainamide, bretylium[7]	See footnote [6]
Cardiac glycoside-induced ventricular tachyarrhythmias[5,8]	Digoxin-immune Fab (digoxin antibody fragments - *Digibind)*	Lidocaine, phenytoin	Self-limited if digoxin is stopped. Phenytoin can also be effective. Avoid DC cardioversion and bretylium, except for ventricular fibrillation or sustained ventricular tachycardia. A beta -blocker or procainamide can make heart block worse.
Torsades de pointes (acquired)	Magnesium sulfate	Cardiac pacing, isoproterenol	Causative agents (e.g., quinidine) should be discontinued. Magnesium sulfate in a dose of 1 g IV, repeated once if necessary, may be effective even in absence of hypomagnesemia. Potassium should be used to raise serum K to between 4 and 5.5 mEq/L[8].

Drugs of Choice for Common Arrhythmias (continued)

1. DC cardioversion is the safest and most effective treatment. For patients with atrial flutter, atrial pacing can also be effective. Patients with Wolff-Parkinson-White syndrome and atrial fibrillation should be treated with IV procainamide if hemodynamically stable and, if not, with DC cardioversion.
2. Vagotonic maneuvers (such as carotid sinus massage, gagging, the Valsalva maneuver, or increasing venous return by straight leg raising) may be tried first.
3. Verapamil and diltiazem are contraindicated for patients receiving intravenous beta-blockers or those with congestive heart failure and should be used with caution in patients taking oral quinidine.
4. DC cardioversion is the safest and most effective treatment. It is preferred by most cardiologists for sustained ventricular tachycardia causing hemodynamic compromise, but some first try a chest thump, IV lidocaine or both.
5. Some ventricular tachycardias can be caused or exacerbated by bradycardia or heart block. In the presence of high-grade heart block, antiarrhythmic drugs can cause cardiac standstill. When high-grade heart block is present, therefore, a temporary pacemaker should be inserted before using antiarrhythmic drugs; pacing may abolish the arrhythmia. When a drug must be used in the presence of heart block, lidocaine is least likely to increase the block.
6. Specialized techniques such as programmed stimulation of the heart may be required to select long-term therapy, and some patients may be candidates for implanted cardioverter/defibrillators (Medical Letter, 36:86, 1994) or radiofrequency catheter ablation (Medical Letter, 38:40, 1996).
7. Defibrillation is the treatment of choice; drugs are for prevention of recurrence.
8. KCl can be given carefully, 10-20 mEq/hr IV, to patients with low or normal serum potassium concentrations. Extreme care must be taken to keep serum potassium below 5.5 mEq/L. In the presence of heart block not associated with paroxysmal atrial tachycardia, potassium should be withheld if the serum concentration is greater than 4.5 mEq/L because high serum potassium may increase atrioventricular block.

Reprinted with permission from reference 30.

Specific Cardiac Dysrhythmias, Principal Causes, and Management (cont)

Dysrhythmia	Cause	Managmeent
Sinus tachycardia	Fever, blood loss, light anesthesia, pain, hypoxia, hypercarbia, catecholamines	Treat cause; propranolol, narcotics, volume expansion, deepen anesthesia
Sinus bradycardia	Normal; deep anesthesia, reflexes, cold, narcotics, sinus node dysfunction	Treat cause, atropine, isoproterenol pacing
Sinus dysrhythmia	Same	Same
Sinus pause or arrest	Beta-blockers, Ca-entry blockers, digitalis excess, sinus dysfunction	Same
SA exit block	Same	Same
Wandering atrial pacemaker dysfunction	Normal; deep anesthesia, sinus	Same
Premature atrial beats	Chronic pulmonary disease, sepsis, myocardial ischemia, central lines	Treat cause; quinidine, procainamide disopyramide if premature atrial beats provoke tachydysrhythmias
Atrial flutter	Organic heart disease, atrial distension, hypertension, pulmonary embolism, metabolic conditions	Treat cause; DC cardioversion, digitalis propranolol, verapamil, quinidine procainamide, disopyramide
Atrial fibrillation	Same	Same
Atrial tachycardia with or without block	Organic heart disease, cor pulmonale, digitalis toxicity	Same as atrial flutter/fibrillation phenytoin if caused by digitalis

Specific Cardiac Dysrhythmias, Principal Causes, and Management

Dysrhythmia	Cause	Management
Multifocal atrial tachycardia	Chronic pulmonary disease, diabetes, coronary artery disease	Same as atrial flutter/fibrillation
AV junctional beats and rhythm	Depressed sinus node function, enhanced automaticity in junctional pacemakers	Atropine, isoproterenol, pacing lidocaine for premature AV junction beats
AV junctional tachycardia	Myocarditis, inferior wall myocardial infarction, open heart surgery, digitalis toxicity	Treat cause; improve hemodynamics consider digitalis if not already digitalized
AV nodal reentrant tachycardia (PSVT)	Stress, anxiety, fatigue, caffeine; occasionally, organic heart disease	Sedation, reassurance, avoid provocative factors; vagal maneuvers, verapamil, edrophonium, propranolol, DC cardioversion, digitalis, antitachycardia pacing
Reentry over a retrograde (concealed) pathway	May account for 30% of cases "routine" PSVT, no specific causes	Quinidine, procainamide, disopyramide otherwise same management for PSVT
Preexcitation syndromes (tachycardia)	Accessory conduction pathways (WPW, LGL, variant)	Same as for reentry over a concealed pathway
Premature ventricular beats (PVB)	Multifactorial, increased prevalence with advanced age	Treat cause, underlying heart disease; lidocaine and all other approved antidysrhythmics, except bretylium
Ventricular tachycardia (VT)	Digitalis toxicity, myocardial ischemia/ infarction, catecholamines, quinidine, disopyramide, procainamide, long Q-T syndrome, and any drugs that prolong Q-T interval	Same as for PVBs; bretylium indicated when VT refractory to other drug management

Dysrhythmia	Cause	Management
Ventricular flutter/ fibrillation	Same causes as for VT	Immediate DC electrical shock, then treat as for VT
1° AV block	Normal; excessive vagal tone, rapid atrial rates, deep anesthesia, narcotics, verapamil, propranolol	Usually none; atropine, isoproterenol
Type I AV block	Same as 1° AV block; organic heart disease, acute inferior wall infarction	Same as for 1° AV block, possibly temporary pacing
Type II AV block	Organic heart disease, acute anterior wall infarction	Atropine and isoproterenol (temporary) pacing (definitive)
Complete AV block	Organic heart disease	Same
Bundle branch and fascicular blocks	Organic heart disease	None; possibly temporary pacing when associated with 1° or type I AV block; pacing when associated with type II AV block

Reproduced with permission from reference 15.

Dosage and Adverse Effects of Some Antiarrhythmic Drugs

Drug	Usual dosage and interval	Effect on ECG	Adverse effects	Serum concentrations#
BETA-ADRENERGIC BLOCKERS				
Propranolol (Inderal, and others)	PO: 10-80 mg q6h (long-acting formulation available) IV: 1-5 mg total (1 mg/min)	Prolongs PR (±) Bradycardia	Fatigue, impotence, heart block, hypotension, heart failure, bronchospasm, depression	Not useful
Acebutolol (Sectral)	PO: 200 mg bid, increase gradually to 600-1200 mg/day	Prolongs PR Sinus bradycardia	Hypotension bradycardia, heart failure bronchospasm, arthritis, myalgia, arthralgia, lupus-like syndrome, pulmonary complications	Not established
Esmolol (Brevibloc)	IV Loading: 500 µg/kg over one minute, followed by 50 µg/kg/min; titrate to desired effect Usual maintenance: 100 µg/kg/min; maximum 300 µg/kg/min	Prolongs PR Sinus bradycardia	Hypotension, heart block, heart failure, bronchospasm, pain at infusion site	0.15 to 2 µg/ml
CALCIUM-CHANNEL BLOCKERS				
Diltiazem (Cardizem)	IV Initial dose: 0.15-0.35 mg/kg (10-25 mg) over 2 min. may be repeated in 15-30 min IV infusion: 5-15 mg/hr	Prolongs PR Sinus bradycardia	Heart block, hypotension, asystole, heart failure, liver damage	Not clinically useful

Drug	Usual dosage and interval	Effect on ECG	Adverse effects	Serum concentrations#
Verapamil HCl (Calan, and others)	IV Initial dose: 5-10 mg over 2-3 min repeat in 15-30 min if necessary IV Infusion: Initial dose is followed by 0.375 mg/min for 30 min IV Maintenance: 0.125 mg/min PO: 40-120 mg tid or qid (long-acting formulation available)	Prolongs PR Sinus bradycardia	Heart block, heart failure, hypotension, asystole, dizziness, headache, fatigue, edema, nausea, constipation	Not clinically useful
QUINIDINE, PROCAINAMIDE, DISOPYRAMIDE				
Quinidine (many manufacturers)	PO (sulfate): 200-400 mg q4-6h PO (gluconate): 324-648 mg q8-12h	Prolongs QRS, QT and (±) PR	Diarrhea and other GI symptoms, cinchonism, hepatic gra necrosis, thrombocytopenia, rashes, hypotension, heart block, tachyarrhythmias, torsades de pointes, fever, lupus-like syndrome	1.5 to 5 μg/ml nulomas and
Procainamide (Pronestyl, and others)	PO: 50-100 mg/kg/day in divided doses q3-4h, q6h (sustained-release), or q12h (Procanbid) IV Loading: 20 mg/min (up to 17 mg/kg) IV Maintenance: 2-4 mg/min	Prolongs QRS, QT and (±) PR	Lupus-like syndrome, confusion, insomnia, GI symptoms, rash, hypotension, arrhythmias, torsades de pointes, blood dyscrasias, fever, hepatitis and hepatic failure, myopathy IV: hypotension, heart block	4 to 10 μg/ml (NAPA active metabolite: 7 to 15 μg/ml)

Dosage and Adverse Effects of Some Antiarrhythmic Drugs (continued)

Drug	Usual dosage and interval	Effect on ECG	Adverse effects	Serum concentrations#
Disopyramide (Norpace, and others)	PO: 100-200 mg q6-8h or 150-300 mg q12h (long-acting formulation)	Prolongs QRS, QT and (±) PR	Anticholinergic effects (urinary retention, aggravation of glaucoma, constipation), hypotension, heart failure, tachyarrhythmias, torsades de pointes, heart block, nausea, vomiting, diarrhea, hypoglycemia, nervousness	2 to 5 μg/ml**
FLECAINIDE, PROPAFENONE, MORICIZINE				
Flecainide (Tambocor)	PO Initial dose: 50-100 mg q12h, increase q4 days (if required) by 50 mg q12h PO Maintenance: ≤ 400 mg/day (≤300 mg for SVT)	Prolongs PR and QRS	Bradycardia, heart block, new ventricular fibrillation, sustained ventricular tachycardia, heart failure, dizziness, blurred vision, nervousness, headache, GI upset, neutropenia	0.2 to 1 μg/ml
Propafenone (Rythmol)	PO Initial dose: 150 mg q8h, increase q3-4 days if required PO Maintenance: 150-300 mg q8h	Prolongs PR and QRS	Bradycardia, heart block, new ventricular fibrillation, sustained ventricular tachycardia, heart failure, dizziness, lightheadedness, metallic taste, bronchospasm, GI upset, hepatic toxicity	Not established due to active metabolites

Drug	Usual dosage and interval	Effect on ECG	Adverse effects	Serum concentrations#
Moricizine (Ethmozine)	PO Initial dose: 200 mg q8h, increase by 150 mg/day q3-4 days if required PO Maintenance: 200-300 mg q8h	Prolongs PR and QRS	Bradycardia, heart failure, new ventricular fibrillation, sustained ventricular tachycardia, nausea, dizziness, headache	Not established
ADENOSINE				
Adenosine (Adenocard)	IV: 6 mg initially; if no conversion after 1-2 minutes, give 12 mg, and repeat once if necessary. Follow each bolus with saline flush.	Prolongs PR Transient heart block	Facial flushing, transient dyspnea, chest discomfort, hypotension; may cause bronchoconstriction in patients with asthma	Not clinically useful
LIDOCAINE AND SIMILAR AGENTS				
Lidocaine (Xylocaine, and others)	IV Loading: 1 mg/kg given over 2 minutes, then 0.5 mg/kg over 2 minutes every 8-10 min x 3 or: 20 mg/min infused over 10 minutes IV Maintenance: 1-4 mg/min	No significant change	Drowsiness or agitation, slurred speech, tinnitus, disorientation, coma, seizures, paresthesias, cardiac depression (especially with excessive accumulation in heart failure or liver failure or infusions for more than 24 hours), bradycardia/asystole	1.5 to 5 μg/ml

Dosage and Adverse Effects of Some Antiarrhythmic Drugs (continued)

Drug	Usual dosage and interval	Effect on ECG	Adverse effects	Serum concentrations#
Tocainide (Tonocard)	PO Initial dose: 200-400 mg q8h with food PO Maintenance: 200-600 mg q8h, maximum 2400 mg/day	No significant change	GI upset, paresthesias, dizziness, tremor, confusion, nightmares, seizures, rash, psychotic reactions, coma, fever, arthralgia, agranulocytosis, aplastic anemia, thrombocytopenia, hepatic granulomas, interstitial pneumonitis	3 to 10 μg/ml
Mexiletine (Mexitil)	PO Initial dose: 150-200 mg q8h taken with food PO Maintenance: 150-300 mg q6-12h, maximum 1200 mg/day	No significant change	GI upset, fatigue, dizziness nervousness, tremor, sleep upset, seizures, psychosis, visual disturbances, fever, blood dyscrasias, hepatitis	0.5 to 2 μg/ml
AMIODARONE, SOTALOL, IBUTILIDE				
Sotalol (Betapace)	PO: 80-160 mg twice daily (Higher doses can be used, but may be associated with increased adverse effects including torsades de pointes)	Prolongs QT, PR Sinus bradycardia	Heart block, hypotension, bronchospasm, bradycardia, torsades de pointes	Generally not clinically useful. 0.5-1.0 1μg/ml for beta-blockade, higher for QT effect

Drug	Usual dosage and interval	Effect on ECG	Adverse effects	Serum concentrations#
Amiodarone (Cordarone)	PO Loading: 800-1600 mg/day for 1-3 weeks, then 600-800 mg/day for 4 weeks PO Maintenance: 100-400 mg/day IV Rapid loading: 150 mg over 10 minutes, which can be repeated once if needed, followed by IV Slow infusion: 360 mg over 6 hours, followed by IV Maintenance: 540 mg over 18 hours	Prolongs PR, QRS and QT Sinus bradycardia	Acute pulmonary toxicity, pulmonary fibrosis, bradycardia, heart block, new ventricular fibrillation, sustained ventricular tachycardia, torsades de pointes (unusual), hyper- or hypothyroidism, GI upset, alcoholic-like hepatitis, peripheral neuropathy, ataxia, tremor, dizziness, photosensitivity, blue-gray skin, corneal microdeposits	1 to 2 μg/ml (usefulness for monitoring toxicity unclear)
Ibutilide (Corvert)	IV: 1 mg over 10 minutes; can be repeated once after 10 minutes if needed	Prolongs QT	Torsades de pointes, AV block	Not clinically useful

Dosage and Adverse Effects of Some Antiarrhythmic Drugs (continued)

Drug	Usual dosage and interval	Effect on ECG	Adverse effects	Serum concentrations#
OTHER AGENTS				
Bretylium (Bretylol, and others; Bretylate in Canada)	IV Loading: 5 mg/kg with additional doses of 10 mg/kg to maximum of 30 mg/kg (effect may be delayed) IV Maintenance: 5-10 mg/kg q6h or continuous infusion 1-2 mg/min	No change Sinus bradycardia	Initial hypertension, orthostatic hypotension, nausea and vomiting, increased sensitivity to catecholamines, initial increase in arrhythmias	Not established
Digoxin (Lanoxin, and others)	IV or PO Loading: 1-1.5 mg over 24 hours in 3-4 divided doses Maintenance: 0.125-0.5 mg/day	Prolongs PR Depresses ST segment Flattens T wave	Bradycardia, AV block, arrhythmias, anorexia, vomiting, diarrhea, nausea, abdominal pain, headache, confusion, abnormal vision	1-2 ng/ml
Magnesium sulfate	IV: 1-2 gm over 5-10 minutes	No change	Areflexia, apnea (very high doses)	Not useful

* Patients with decreased hepatic or renal function may require lower dosage.

#Range of usually effective and tolerated concentrations

** Not reliable due to saturable protein binding

Reprinted with permission from reference 30.

Pharmacology

Local Anesthetics

Pharmacologic and Clinical Characteristics of Local Anesthetics

Characteristic	Procaine (Novocaine)	Chloroprocaine (Nesacaine)	Lidocaine (Xylocaine)	Prilocaine (Citanest)	Mepivacaine (Carbocaine)	Bupivacaine (Marcaine)	Tetracaine (Pontocaine)	Etidocaine (Duracaine)
Physicochemical								
Potency ratio*	1	2	3	3	3	15	15	15
Toxicity ratio*	1	0.75	1.5	1.5	2.0	10	12	10
Anesthetic index (1)	1	3	3	2	1.5	1.5	1.25	1.5
pH of plain solution	5 - 6.5	2.7 - 4	6.5	4.5	4.5	4.5 - 6	4.5 - 6.5	4.5
pKa	8.9	8.7	7.9	7.7	7.6	8.1	8.6	7.7
Clinical								
Latency	Moderate	Fast	Fast	Fast	Fast	Moderate	Very slow	Fast
Penetrance	Moderate	Marked	Marked	Marked	Moderate	Moderate	Poor	Moderate
Duration	Short	Very short	Intermediate	Intermediate	Intermediate	Long	Long	Long
Duration ratio*	1	0.75	1.5 - 2	1.75 - 2	2 - 2.5	6 - 8	6 - 8	5 - 8

Pharmacologic and Clinical Characteristics of Local Anesthetics

Characteristic	Procaine (Novocaine)	Chloroprocaine (Nesacaine)	Lidocaine (Xylocaine)	Prilocaine (Citanest)	Mepivacaine (Carbocaine)	Bupivacaine (Marcaine)	Tetracaine (Pontocaine)	Etidocaine (Duracaine)
Concentration of Solution (%)								
Local infiltration	0.5	0.5	0.25 - 0.5	0.25 - 0.5	0.25 - 0.5	0.125 - 0.25	0.1 - 0.15	0.5 - 0.2
Regional IV	1	1	0.5	0.5	0.5	0.125 - 0.25	0.1 - 0.15	0.15 - 0.2
Small nerve sympathetic block	1	1	0 5	0.5	0.5	0.25	0.25	0.25
Block of large nerve or plexus	2	2	1 - 1.5	1 - 2	1 - 15	0.375 - 0.5	0.15 - 0.3	0.5 - 1
Extradural block								
Analgesia	1.5	1.5	1	1	1	0.25 - 0.375	0.2- - 0.4	0.5 - 1.0
Motor block	3	3	2	2	2	0.5 - 0.75	0.3 - 0.5	1 - 1.5
Maximum single dose (mg/kg)	15	15	7	8	7	3	2.5	4

Procaine used as standard of reference = l; ratios vary according to techniques of regional anesthesia used. Anesthetic index = potency ratio/toxicity ratio.

Reprinted with permission from reference 31.

Comparable Safe Doses of Local Anesthetics (mg/kg)*

	Areas Injected			
		Central Blocks‡		
Drugs	Peripheral blocks¥	Plain	With Epi 1:200,000	Intercostal Blocks§ with Epi 1:200,000
2-Chloroprocaine	-	20	25	-
Procaine	-	14	18	-
Lidocaine	20	7	9	6
Mepivacaine	20	7	9	6
Bupivacaine	5	2	2	2
Tetracaine	-	2	2	-

*Estimated to produce peak plasma levels that are less than half the plasma levels at which seizures could occur.

‡Areas of moderate vascularity (i.e. caudal epidural blocks).

¥Areas of low vascularity (i.e., axillary blocks using local anesthetic solutions containing 1:200,000 epinephrine).

§Areas of high vascularity (i.e., intercostal blocks using local anesthetic solutions containing 1:200,000 epinephrine).

Reprinted with permission from reference 32.

Local Anesthetics Used for Spinal Anesthesia

Agent	Concentration	Usual Adult Dose	Baricity	Usual Duration (min)
Lidocaine	5% in 7.5% glucose	50 - 100 mg (1 - 2 ml)	Hyperbaric	45 - 80
	2%	40 - 60 mg (2 - 3 ml)	Isobaric	60 - 100
Bupivacaine	0.75% in 8.25% glucose	9 - 15 mg (1.2 - 2 ml)	Hyperbaric	90 - 240
	0.5%	15 mg (3 ml)	Isobaric	90 - 240
Tetracaine	0.5% in 5% glucose	10 - 20 mg (2 - 4 ml)	Hyperbaric	150 - 300
	0.5%	10 - 20 mg (2 - 4 ml)	Isobaric	
	0.1%	10 mg (10 ml)	Hypobaric	

Local Anesthetics Used for Epidural Anesthesia

Agent	Concentration (%)	Maximum Adult Dose Plain Solution	With Epinephrine	Duration (min)
Chloroprocaine	2 - 3	≤800 mg (40 ml 2%)	≤900 mg (30 ml 3%)	30 - 75
Lidocaine	1 - 2	≤300 mg (30 ml 1%)	≤500 mg (50 ml 1%)	50 - 120
Mepivacaine	1 - 2	≤300 mg (30 ml 1%)	≤500 mg (50 ml 1%)	60 - 150
Bupivacaine	0.25 - 0.75	≤175 mg (35 ml 0.5%)	≤225 mg (45 ml 0.5%)	120 - 240

Reprinted with permission from reference 33.

Central Neural Blockade for Acute Pain Management in Children*

Block	Drug recommended	Dose (mg/kg)	Duration (hours)	Notes
Lumbar epidural: single dose	1 - 1.5% lidocaine	7 - 9	1 - 2	Use 1 - 1.5 mL/blocked segment
	0.25% bupivacaine	1.5 - 2.5	4 - 8	
	0.125% bupivacaine	1.5 - 2.5	2 - 4	
	Preservative-free morphine	0.05 - 0.1 Max: 5 mg	8 - 24	May cause respiratory depression
Lumbar epidural: continuous infusion	0.125% bupivacaine	0.3 mL/kg/h	NA	Fentanyl has much less rostral spread than morphine
	0.1% bupivacaine + fentanyl 2 μg/mL	0.3 mL/kg/h	NA	
Caudal epidural: single dose	1 - 1.5% lidocaine	7 - 9	1 - 2	1 mL/kg of local agent is required for T6 - T8 block
	0.25% bupivacaine	1.5 - 2.5	4 - 8	
	0.125% bupivacaine	1.5 - 2.5	2 - 4	
	Preservative-free morphine	0.05 - 0.1 Max 5 mg	8 - 24	

Block	Drug recommended	Dose (mg/kg)	Duration (hours)	Notes
Caudal epidural: continuous infusion	0.25% bupivacaine	0.3 mL/kg/h	NA	Some motor block will occur with 0.25% bupivacaine
	0.1% bupivacaine + fentanyl 2 μg/mL	0.3 mL/kg/h	NA	
Thoracic epidural: single dose	1 - 1.5% lidocaine	7 - 9	1 - 2	0.5 - 0.7 mL of local anesthetic is needed per segment blocked
	0.25% bupivacaine	1.5 - 2.5	4 - 8	
	0.125% bupivacaine	1.5 - 2.5	2 - 4	
Thoracic epidural: continuous infusion	0.125% bupivacaine	0.2 mL/kg/h	NA	
	0. 1% bupivacaine + fentanyl 2 μg/mL	0.2 mL/kg/h	NA	

* Recommendations for children over 6 months of age.

Reprinted with permission from reference 20.

Recommended Doses of Local Anesthetic for Peripheral Neural Blockade in Children

Block	Agent	Dose	Notes
Intercostal	1 - 1.5% lidocaine with epinephrine 1:200,000	1 - 3 mL/level	Highest systemic drug levels
	0.25% Bupivacaine with epinephrine 1:200,000	1 - 3 mL/level	
Intrapleural	0.25% Bupivacaine with epinephrine 1:200,000	0.4 mL/kg	
	1 - 1.5% lidocaine with epinephrine 1 :200,000	0.4 mL/kg	
Femoral	0.25% bupivacaine with epinephrine 1:200,000	0.4 mL/kg	Max 10 mL
Penile (ring block)	0.25% Bupivacaine	1 - 8 mL	Avoid the use of epinephrine

Reprinted with permission from reference 20.

Recommended Volumes of Anesthetic Solution for Peripheral Blocks for Children

	Recommended Volume of Anesthetic Solution According to the Weight of Children				Total Volume
Site of Block	**<20 kg**	**20 - 29 kg**	**30 - 45 kg**	**>45 kg**	**(ml/kg)**
Supraclavicular/ interscalene block	0.5 - 1 ml/kg	15 - 20 ml	20 - 22.5 ml	22.5 - 25 ml	0.25
Axillary block	0.3 - 0.6 ml/kg	10 - 15 ml	13 - 18 ml	18 - 20 ml	0.33
Femoral nerve block	0.5 ml/kg	10 - 12.5 ml	12.5 - 15 ml	15 - 17.5 ml	0.30
Sciatic nerve block	0.5 ml/kg	10 - 12.5 ml	12.5 - 15 ml	15 - 17.5 ml	0.15 - 0.2

Reprinted with permission from reference 33.

Pharmacology

Drug Infusions

Drug Infusion Calculations

$$I = \frac{0.6 \times V \times W \times R}{D}$$

Where:
- I = Infusion rate in ml/hr
- V = volume of infusion in ml
- W = weight of patient
- R = Rate required in µg/kg/min
- D = Drug dose added to infusion

Drug Infusions

Dopamine - 200 mg/250 ml

	ml/hr for a given weight (kg)						
µg/kg/min	**10**	**50**	**60**	**70**	**80**	**90**	**100**
1	0.8	4	5	5	6	7	8
2	1.5	8	9	11	12	14	15
3	2.3	11	14	16	18	20	23
4	3.0	15	18	21	24	27	30
5	3.8	19	23	26	30	34	38

Dobutamine - 250 mg/250 ml

	ml/hr for a given weight (kg)						
µg/kg/min	**10**	**50**	**60**	**70**	**80**	**90**	**100**
2	1.2	6	7	8	10	11	12
3	1.8	9	11	13	14	16	18
5	3.0	15	18	21	24	27	30
10	6.0	30	36	42	48	54	60
15	9.0	45	54	63	72	81	90

Epinephrine - 1 mg/250 ml

	ml/hr for a given weight (kg)						
µg/kg/min	**10**	**50**	**60**	**70**	**80**	**90**	**100**
0.01	1.5	8	9	11	12	14	15
0.03	4.5	23	27	32	36	41	45
0.05	7.5	38	45	53	60	68	75
0.10	15	75	90	105	120	135	150
0.15	22.5	113	135	158	180	203	225

Isoproterenol - 1 mg/250 ml

	ml/hr for a given weight (kg)						
µg/kg/min	**10**	**50**	**60**	**70**	**80**	**90**	**100**
0.01	1.5	8	9	11	12	14	15
0.03	4.5	23	27	32	36	41	45
0.05	7.5	38	45	53	60	68	75
0.10	15	75	90	105	120	135	150
0.15	22.5	113	135	158	180	203	225

Lidocaine - 1 gm/250 ml

	ml/hr for a given weight (kg)						
µg/kg/min	**10**	**50**	**60**	**70**	**80**	**90**	**100**
10	1.5	8	9	11	12	14	15
20	3.0	15	18	21	24	27	30
30	4.5	23	27	32	36	41	45
40	6.0	30	36	42	48	54	60

Nitroglycerin - 50 mg/250 ml

	ml/hr for a given weight (kg)						
µg/kg/min	**10**	**50**	**60**	**70**	**80**	**90**	**100**
0.25	0.75	4	5	5	6	7	8
0.5	1.5	8	9	11	12	14	15
1.0	3.0	15	18	21	24	27	30
2.0	6.0	30	36	42	48	54	60

Drug Infusions (continued)

Nitroprusside - 50 mg/250 ml

		ml/hr for a given weight (kg)					
µg/kg/min	**10**	**50**	**60**	**70**	**80**	**90**	**100**
0.25	0.75	4	5	5	6	7	8
0.5	1.5	8	9	11	12	14	15
1.0	3.0	15	18	21	24	27	30
2.0	6.0	30	36	42	48	54	60

Norepinephrine - 4 mg/250 ml

		ml/hr for a given weight (kg)					
µg/kg/min	**10**	**50**	**60**	**70**	**80**	**90**	**100**
0.1	3.75	19	23	26	30	34	38
0.2	7.5	38	45	53	60	68	75
0.3	11.25	56	68	79	90	101	113
0.4	15.0	75	90	105	120	135	150

Phentolamine - 20 mg/250 ml

		ml/hr for a given weight (kg)					
µg/kg/min	**10**	**50**	**60**	**70**	**80**	**90**	**100**
0.5	3.75	19	23	26	30	34	38
1.0	7.5	38	45	53	60	68	75
2.0	15	75	90	105	120	135	150
3.0	22.5	113	135	158	180	203	225

Phenylephrine - 10 mg/250 ml

µg/kg/min	10	50	60	70	80	90	100
	ml/hr for a given weight (kg)						
0.05	0.8	4	5	5	6	7	8
0.10	1.5	8	9	11	12	14	15
0.15	2.3	11	14	16	18	20	23
0.20	3.0	15	18	21	24	27	30

Procainamide - 2 gm/250 ml

µg/kg/min	10	50	60	70	80	90	100
	ml/hr for a given weight (kg)						
10	0.75	4	5	5	6	7	8
20	1.5	8	9	11	12	14	15
50	3.75	19	23	26	30	34	38

Physiology / Pathophysiology

Airway Management / Respiratory System

Suggested Contents of the Portable Storage Unit for Difficult Airway Management

IMPORTANT: The items listed in this table represent suggestions. The contents of the portable storage unit should be customized to meet the specific needs, preferences, and skills of the practitioner and health-care facility.

1. Rigid laryngoscope blades of alternate design and size from those routinely used.
2. Endotracheal tubes of assorted size.
3. Endotracheal tube guides. Examples include (but are not limited to) semirigid stylets with or without a hollow core for jet ventilation, light wands, and forceps designed to manipulate the distal portion of the endotracheal tube.
4. Fiberoptic intubation equipment.
5. Retrograde intubation equipment.
6. At least one device suitable for emergency nonsurgical airway ventilation. Examples include (but are not limited to) a transtracheal jet ventilator, a hollow jet ventilation stylet, the laryngeal mask, and the esophageal-tracheal combitube.
7. Equipment suitable for emergency surgical airway access (e.g., cricothyrotomy).
8. An exhaled CO_2 detector.

Reproduced with permission from reference 34.

American Society of Anesthesiologists Difficult Airway Algorithm

1. Assess the likelihood and clinical impact of basic management problems:
   - A. Difficult intubation
   - B. Difficult ventilation
   - C. Difficulty with patient cooperation or consent

2. Consider the relative merits and feasibility of basic management choices:
   - A. Non-Surgical Technique for Initial Approach to Intubation vs. Surgical Technique for Initial Approach to Intubation
   - B. Awake Intubation vs. Intubation Attempts After Induction of General Anesthesia
   - C. Preservation of Spontaneous Ventilation vs. Ablation of Spontaneous Ventilation

3. Develop primary and alternative strategies:

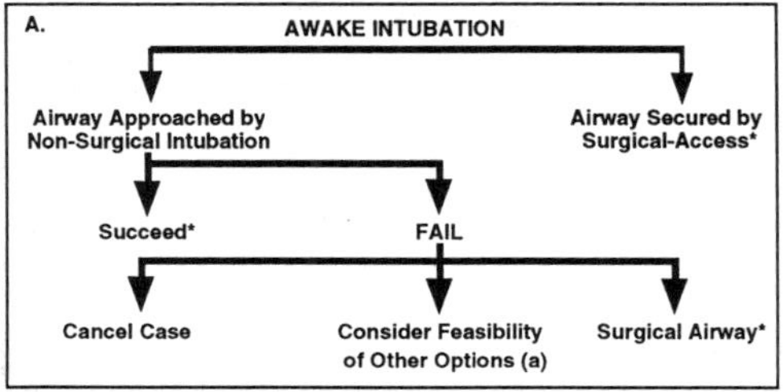

A. AWAKE INTUBATION

Airway Approached by Non-Surgical Intubation

Airway Secured by Surgical-Access*

Succeed*

FAIL

Cancel Case

Consider Feasibility of Other Options (a)

Surgical Airway*

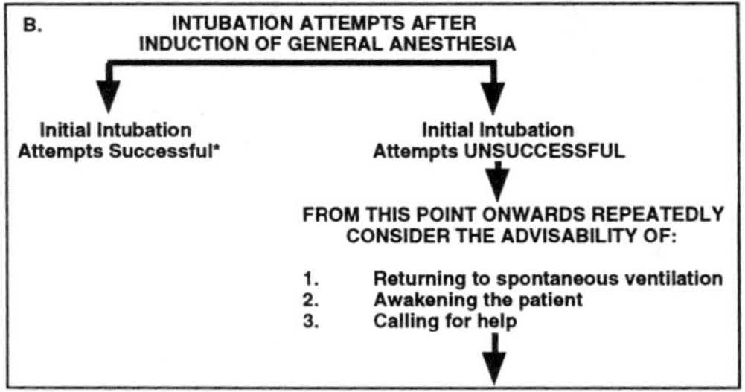

B. INTUBATION ATTEMPTS AFTER INDUCTION OF GENERAL ANESTHESIA

Initial Intubation Attempts Successful*

Initial Intubation Attempts UNSUCCESSFUL

FROM THIS POINT ONWARDS REPEATEDLY CONSIDER THE ADVISABILITY OF:

1. Returning to spontaneous ventilation
2. Awakening the patient
3. Calling for help

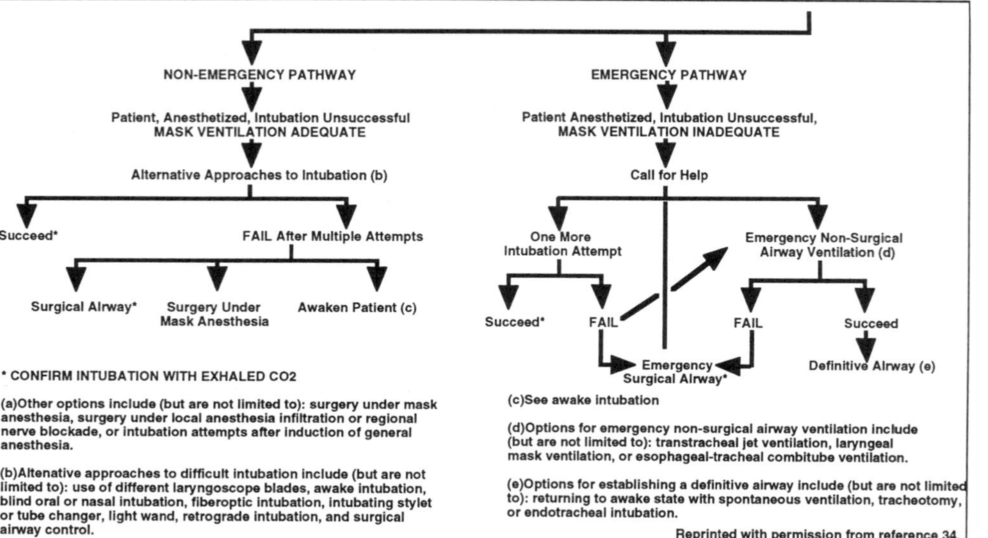
NON-EMERGENCY PATHWAY
Patient, Anesthetized, Intubation Unsuccessful
MASK VENTILATION ADEQUATE
Alternative Approaches to Intubation (b)
Succeed*
FAIL After Multiple Attempts
Surgical Airway*
Surgery Under Mask Anesthesia
Awaken Patient (c)
EMERGENCY PATHWAY
Patient Anesthetized, Intubation Unsuccessful,
MASK VENTILATION INADEQUATE
Call for Help
One More Intubation Attempt
Emergency Non-Surgical Airway Ventilation (d)
Succeed*
FAIL
FAIL
Succeed
Emergency Surgical Airway*
Definitive Airway (e)
* CONFIRM INTUBATION WITH EXHALED CO2
(a)Other options include (but are not limited to): surgery under mask anesthesia, surgery under local anesthesia infiltration or regional nerve blockade, or intubation attempts after induction of general anesthesia.
(b)Altenative approaches to difficult intubation include (but are not limited to): use of different laryngoscope blades, awake intubation, blind oral or nasal intubation, fiberoptic intubation, intubating stylet or tube changer, light wand, retrograde intubation, and surgical airway control.
(c)See awake intubation
(d)Options for emergency non-surgical airway ventilation include (but are not limited to): transtracheal jet ventilation, laryngeal mask ventilation, or esophageal-tracheal combitube ventilation.
(e)Options for establishing a definitive airway include (but are not limited to): returning to awake state with spontaneous ventilation, tracheotomy, or endotracheal intubation.
Reprinted with permission from reference 34.

Indications for Endotracheal Intubation

1. Protection of the airway
2. Upper airway obstruction
3. Facilitation of bronchial hygiene
4. Positive pressure ventilation (includes continuous positive end expiratory pressure (CPAP or PEEP))
5. Surgical field considerations

These indications can also serve as guidelines to extubation.

Definitions Regarding the Difficult Airway

Difficult airway

- A conventionally trained anesthetist experiences difficulty with mask ventilation, endotracheal intubation, or both.

Difficult mask ventilation

- It is not possible for the unassisted anesthesiologist to maintain SaO_2 >90% using 100% O_2 and positive pressure mask ventilation in a patient whose SaO_2 was > 90% before anesthetic intervention.
- It is not possible for the unassisted anesthesiologist to prevent or reverse causes of inadequate ventilation during positive mask ventilation.

Difficult laryngoscopy

- It is not possible to visualize any portion of the vocal cords with conventional laryngoscopy.

Difficult endotracheal intubation

- Proper insertion of the endotracheal tube with conventional laryngoscopy requires more than three attempts or more than 10 minutes.

Reproduced with permission from reference 34.

Anatomic Factors Relevant to Difficult Intubation

Anatomic factors relevant to difficult intubation. At laryngoscopy the line of vision in the cords must be cleared. Difficulty may occur if: (1) cords, (2) upper teeth, or (3) tongue, are displaced in the direction of the arrows Even with no pathology this may occur due to variation in the normal anatomy.

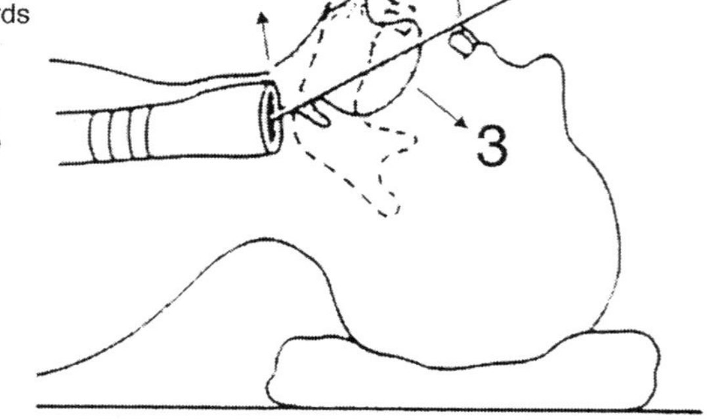

Reprinted with permission from reference 35.

Mallampati Classification of the Airway

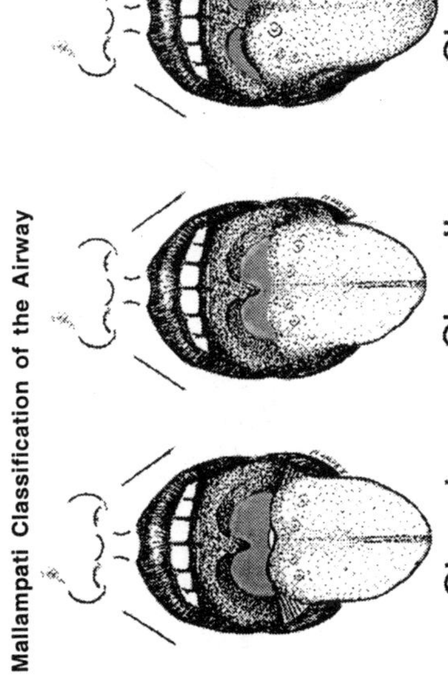

Class I
Soft palate, tonsillar fauces, tonsillar pillars and uvula visualized

Class II
Soft palate, tonsillar fauces, and uvula visualized

Class III
Soft palate and base of the uvula visualized

Class IV
Soft palate not visualized

Modified with permission from reference 36.

Anatomic Causes and Mechanisms of Difficult Laryngoscopy

Cause	Example(s)	Primary mechanism
1. Disproportion	Mallampati class III airway Pierre robin syndrome Down Syndrome	Disproportionately increased size of the base of tongue
	Receding chin Very short thyromental distance Very short hyomental distance	Larynx relatively anterior to the rest of the upper airway structures
2. Distortion		
From intrinsic factors	Carcinoma of larynx Laryngeal edema	Stenosis and deviation from intrinsic or extrinsic factors or both
From extrinsic factors	Goiter Carcinoma of the base of tongue Postoperative hematoma in the neck	
3. Decreased mobility of joints	Klippel-Feil syndrome Ankylosing spondylitis Rheumatoid arthritis	Impedance of axis alignment
4. Dentition overbite	Likely to be a significant factor particularly in association with Mallampati class II and class III airway	Impedance of axis alignment

Reproduced with permission from reference 37.

Laryngoscopic View Grading System

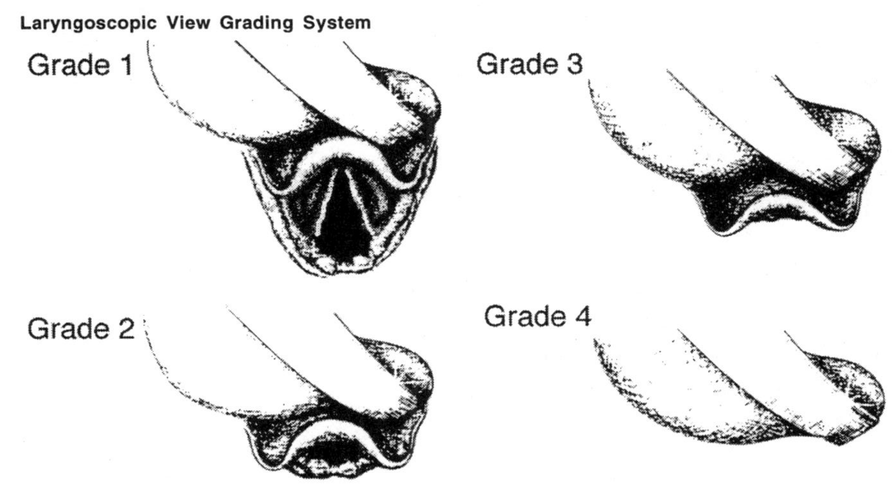

Modified with permission from reference 35.

Visualization of Glottitis During Laryngoscopy

Grade	Approximate Frequency	View
1	99%	Glottis (including anterior and posterior commissures) could be fully exposed.
2	1%	Glottis could be partly exposed (anterior commissure not visualized).
3	0.05%	Glottis could not be exposed (corniculate cartilages only could be visualized).
4	0.001%	Glottis including corniculate cartilage could not be exposed.

Grades 1 and 2 are considered "adequate exposure" and grades 3 and 4 "inadequate exposure".

Airway Compromising Conditions

Group	Pathologic condition	Principal pathologic/clinical features
I. Congenital:	A. *Supralaryngeal*	
	1. Pierre Robin syndrome	Micrognathia, macroglossia, cleft soft palate
	2. Treacher Collins syndrome	Auricular and ocular defects; malar and mandibular hypoplasia; outgrows
	3. Goldenhar's syndrome	Auricular and ocular defects; malar and mandibular hypoplasia; occipitalization of atlas; does not outgrow
	4. Down syndrome	Poorly developed or absent bridge of the nose; macroglossia
	5. Klippel-Feil syndrome	Congenital fusion of a variable number of cervical vertebrae; restriction of neck movement
	B. *Sublaryngeal*	
	1. Goiter	Compression of trachea, deviation of larynx-trachea
II. Acquired:	A. *Infections*	
	1. Supraglottitis	Laryngeal edema
	2. Croup	Laryngeal edema
	3. Abscess (intraoral, retropharyngeal)	Distortion of the airway and trismus
	4. Ludwig's angina	Distortion of the airway and trismus
	B. *Arthritis*	
	1. Rheumatoid arthritis	Temporomandibular joint ankylosis, cricoarytenoid arthritis, deviation of larynx, restricted mobility of cervical spine

2. Ankylosing spondylitis	Ankylosis of cervical spine; less commonly, ankylosis of temporomandibular joints; lack of mobility of cervical spine
C. *Benign tumors*	Stenosis or distortion of the airway
1. Ex: cystic hygroma, lipoma, adenoma, goiter	
D. *Malignant tumors*	Stenosis or distortion of the airway; fixation of larynx or adjacent tissues secondary to infiltration or fibrosis from irradiation
1. Ex: Carcinoma of tongue, carcinoma of larynx, carcinoma of thyroid	
E. *Trauma*	Edema of the airway, hematoma, unstable fracture(s) of the maxillae, mandible, and cervical vertebrae
1. Ex: Facial injury, cervical spine injury, laryngeal-tracheal trauma	
F. *Obesity*	Short, thick neck; redundant tissue in the oropharynx; sleep apnea
G. *Acromegaly*	Macroglossia; prognathism
H. *Acute burns*	Edema of airway

Reproduced with permission from reference 37.

Congenital Syndromes and Hereditary Diseases Associated with Difficult Airway

Micrognathia and mandibular hypoplasia

- Carpenter's syndrome
- Christ-Siemens-Touraine syndrome
- Cri du chat syndrome
- DiGeorge syndrome
- Edwards' syndrome (trisomy 18)
- Goldenhar's syndrome
- King-Denborough syndrome
- Letterer-Sewe disease
- Meckel's syndrome
- Mobius' syndrome
- Noonan's syndrome
- Osteochondrodystrophies (dwarfism)
- Patau syndrome (trisomy 13)
- Pierre Robin syndrome
- Smith-Lemli-Opitz syndrome
- Treacher Collins syndrome
- Turner's syndrome

Macroglossia

- Beckwith-Wiedemann syndrome
- Down syndrome (trisomy 21)
- Farber's disease
- Hurler's syndrome (mucopolysaccharidosis, type I)
- Pompe's disease (glycogen storage disease, type II)

Cervical instability or limited cervical mobility

- Arnold-Chiari malformation
- Down syndrome (see Macroglossia)
- Hurler's syndrome (see Macroglossia)
- Klippel-Feil syndrome
- Larsen's syndrome
- Marfan syndrome
- Maroteaux-Lamy syndrome (mucopolysaccharidosis, type VI)
- Morquio's syndrome (mucopolysaccharidosis, type IV)
- Osteochondrodystrophies (dwarfism)

Syndromes affecting temporomandibular joint and limited mouth opening

Arthrogryposis
Behcet's syndrome
Cockayne-Touraino syndrome (dystrophic epidermolysis bullae)
CREST syndrome
Epidermolysis bullosum
Freeman-Sheldon syndrome (whistling face)
Juvenile rheumatoid arthritis (Still's disease)
Myositis ossificans
Scleroderma
Treacher Collins syndrome

Midface hypoplasia and prominent or abnormal mandible

Andersen's syndrome
Apert's syndrome
Crouzon syndrome
Hallermann-Streiff syndrome
Oral-facial-digital syndrome
Pfeiffer's syndrome
Rieger's syndrome

Obstructing mass

Cherubism (tumors)
Encephalocele
Farber's disease (tumors of larynx; see Macroglossia)
Kasabach-Merritt syndrome (hemangioma)
Letterer-Siwe disease (laryngeal fibrosis; see Micrognathia)
Neurofibromatosis (fibroma)
Stevens-Johnson syndrome (bullae)
Sturge-Weber syndrome (hemangioma)

Enlarged mandible or distortion of facial features

Gaucher disease
Maroteaux-Lamy syndrome
Morquio's syndrome
Pyle's disease
Saethre-Chotzen syndrome
Sanfilippo's syndrome (mucopolysaccharidosis, type III)
Sotos' syndrome (cerebral gigantism)

Reproduced with permission from reference 37.

Anomalies According to Anatomic Location

(with special emphasis on the difficult pediatric airway)

I. Head Anomalies
   A. Mass lesions
      1. Encephalocele
      2. Soft tissue sarcoma
   B. Gross enlargement (macrocephaly)
      1. Severe hydrocephaly
      2. Mucopolysaccharidosis [Hurler's syndrome]
   C. Disease affecting access to the airway
      1. Certain conjoined twins [thoracopagus]
      2. Presence of a head stereotactic frame

II. Facial anomalies
   A. Maxillary and mandibular disease
      1. Maxillary hypoplasia
         a. Apert's syndrome
         b. Crouzon's disease
      2. Mandibular hypoplasia and hyperplasia
         a. Pierre Robin syndrome
         b. Treacher Collins syndrome
         c. Goldenhar's syndrome
   B. Temporomandibular joint disease
      1. Reduced mobility
      2. Ankylosis (traumatic, congenital, inflammatory, infectious)

III. Mouth and tongue anomalies
   A. Microstomia
      1. Congenital (whistling face syndrome)
      2. Acquired (burns, chemical injection)
   B. Tongue disease
      1. Enlargement
         a. Beckwith-Wiedemann syndrome
         b. Down syndrome
         c. Congenital hypothyroidism
         d. Pompe's disease
      2. Swelling
         a. After surgery
         b. Burn injury
         c. Trauma
         d. Ludwig's angina
      3. Tumors
         a. Hemangioma
         b. Lymphangioma

- IV. Nasal, palatal, and pharyngeal anomalies
  - A. Nasal anomalies
    1. Choanal atresia
    2. Masses
       - a. Encephaloceles
       - b. Gliomas
       - c. Foreign body
  - B. Palatal anomalies
    1. Arch anomaly
    2. Cleft palate
    3. Swelling
    4. Hematoma
  - C. Pharynx
    1. Enlarged adenoids
    2. Enlarged tonsils
    3. Others (tumors, peritonsillar abscess)
  - D. Pharyngeal wall
    1. Retropharyngeal and parapharyngeal abscess
    2. Pharyngeal bullae or scarring
       - a. Epidermolysis bullosa
       - b. Erythema multiforme bullosum
- V. Laryngeal anomalies
  - A. Supraglottic disease
    1. Laryngomalacia
    2. Epiglottitis
  - B. Glottic disease
    1. Congenital lesions
       - a. Vocal cord paralysis
       - b. Laryngeal web, cyst, and laryngocele
    2. Papillomatosis
    3. Granuloma formation
    4. Foreign body (see Tracheal and bronchial anomalies)
  - C. Subglottic disease
    1. Congenital stenosis
    2. Infectious (croup)
    3. Inflammatory disease
       - a. Edema
       - b. Traumatic stenosis

VI. Tracheal and bronchial anomalies
   A. Tracheobronchial tree
      1. Tracheomalacia
      2. Croup
      3. Bacterial tracheitis
      4. Mediastinal masses
      5. Vascular malformations
      6. Foreign body aspiration
      7. Others
         a Tracheal stenosis
         b. Webbing
         c. Fistula
         d. Diverticulum

VII. Neck and spine anomalies
   A. Neck
      1. Masses
         a. Lymphatic malformation
         b. Hemangioma
         c. Teratoma
      2. Skin contracture
         a. After burn
         b. Inflammatory
            i. Scleroderma
            ii. Epidermolysis bullosa
            iii. Erythema multiforme bullosum
   B. Spine
      1. Limited cervical spine mobility
         a. Congenital disease (Klippel-Fiel syndrome)
         b. Acquired disease
            i. Surgery (fusion)
            ii. Trauma (vertebral fracture)
            iii. Inflammatory disease (juvenile rheumatoid arthritis)
      2. Cervical spine instability
         a. Congenital disease (Down syndrome)
         b. Acquired disease
            i. Trauma (subluxation, fracture)
            ii. Inflammatory disease (juvenile rheumatoid arthritis)

Reproduced with permission from reference 37.

Techniques for Difficult Airway Management

IMPORTANT: This table displays commonly cited techniques. It is not a comprehensive list. The order of presentation is alphabetical and does not imply preference for a given technique or sequence of use. Combinations of techniques may be employed. The techniques chosen by the practitioner in a particular case will depend upon specific needs, preferences, skills, and clinical constraints.

1. Techniques for difficult intubation

Alternative laryngoscope blades
Awake intubation
Blind intubation (oral or nasal)
Fiberoptic intubation
Intubating stylets/tube changer
Light wand
Retrograde intubation
Surgical airway access

2. Techniques for difficult ventilation

Esophageal-tracheal combitube
Intratracheal jet stylet
Laryngeal mask
Oral and nasopharyngeal airways
Rigid ventilating bronchoscope
Surgical airway access
Transtracheal jet ventilation
Two-person mask ventilation

Reproduced with permission from reference 39.

Signs of Tracheal Intubation

Non-fail-safe signs

1. Breath sounds over chest
2. No breath sounds over stomach
3. No gastric distention
4. Chest rise and fall
5. Intercostal spaces filling out during inspiration
6. Large spontaneous exhaled tidal volumes
7. Respiratory gas moisture disappearing on inhalation and reappearing on exhalation
8. Hearing air exit from the endotracheal tube when the chest is compressed
9. Reservoir bag having the appropriate compliance
10. Reciprocating pulsed pressures to and from suprasternal notch and to and from balloon on the pilot tube of the endotracheal tube
11. Progressive arterial desaturation by pulse oximetry

Near fail-safe signs

1. Carbon dioxide excretion waveform
2. Rapid expansion of a tracheal indicator bulb

Fail-safe signs

1. Endotracheal tube visualized between vocal cords
2. Fiberoptic visualization of cartilaginous rings of the trachea and tracheal carina

Reproduced with permission from reference 37.

Objective Quantitative Criteria for Tracheal Intubation

Category	Variable	Acceptable range	Possible intubation chest PT, oxygen, drugs, close monitoring	Probable intubation and ventilation
Mechanics	Vital capacity (ml/kg)	67 - 75	65 - 15	< 15
	Inspiratory force (ml H_2O)	100 - 50	50 - 25	< 25
Oxygenation	$A\text{-}aDO_2$ (mm Hg) room air	< 38	38 - 55	> 55
	$FiO_2 = 1.0$	<100	100 - 450	>450
	PaO_2 (mm Hg)			
	room air	> 72	72-55	< 55
	$FiO_2 = 1.0$	>400	400 - 200	<200
Ventilation	Respiratory rate, (breaths/min)	10 - 25	25 - 40 or <8	>40 or <6
	$PaCO_2$ (mm Hg)	35 - 45	45 - 60	> 60

PT, physical therapy; $A\text{-}aDO_2$, alveolar-arterial partial pressure of oxygen difference; PaO_2 and $PaCO_2$, arterial partial pressure of oxygen and carbon dioxide, respective; FiO_2, inspired concentration of oxygen.

Modified with permission from reference 38.

Relevant Diameters of the Different Sizes of Laryngeal Mask Airways (LMA), Endotracheal Tubes (ETT), and Fiberoptic Bronchoscopes (FOB) That Fit Into the ETTs

LMA Size	Patient Weight (kg)	LMA ID (mm)	Cuff Volume (ml)	Largest ETT inside LMA (ID, mm)	Largest FOB inside ETT (mm)	Type of FOB That Will Pass through ETT
1	<5	5.25	2 - 5	3.5	2.7	Olympus PF-27M, ENF-P2, BF-N20; Pentax FB-10H, FI-10P
2	10 - 20	7.0	7 - 10	4.5	3.5	Olympus ENF-P3, BF-3C20; Pentax FNL-15S
2.5	20 - 30	8.4	14	5.0	4.0	Olympus LF-1, LF-2
3	30 - 70	10	15 - 20	6.0 cuffed	5.0	Olympus BF-2TR, BF-P20D
4	>70	10	25 - 30	6.0 cuffed	5.0	Pentax FB-19H, FB-19H3
5	>90	11.5	35 - 40	7.0 cuffed	6.5	Many brands

Adapted with permission from reference 39.

Relevant Length of Laryngeal Mask Airway (LMA) and Endotracheal Tubes (ETT)

LMA Size	Patient Weight (kg)	Length from Proximal Edge of LMA Adaptor to Grille (cm)	Largest ETT (ID, mm)	Length of Largest ETT from Distal Edge of ETT Adaptor to ETT Tip (0.5 cm of male end of ETT adaptor is outside of ETT lumen (cm))	Distance Tip of ETT Protrudes from Grille When Distal Edge of ETT Adaptor Is Flush Against the Proximal Edge of the LMA Adaptor (cm)
1	<5	10.5	3.5	18.5	8.0
2	10 - 20	14.5	4.5	23	8.5
2.5	20 - 30	15.5	5.0	28	12.5
3	30 - 70	20.0	6.0 cuffed	29	9.0*
4	>70	20.0	6.0 cuffed	29	9.0*
5	>90	22.0	7.0 cuffed	29	9.0*

*Proximal border of ETT cuff to tip of ETT = 4.5 - 5.0 cm.

Adapted with permission from reference 39.

Laryngeal Mask Airways

Patient Size	Mask Size	Maximum Cuff Inflation (mL)	Standard LMA ID (mm)	Standard Tube Length (cm)	LMA-Flexible™ ID (mm)	LMA-Flexible™ Tube Length (cm)
Neonates/infants up to 5 kg	1	5	5.25	11.5	Not available	Not available
Infants between 5 - 10 kg	1.5	7	6.1	13.5	Not available	Not available
Infants/children between 10 - 20 kg	2	10	7.0	15.5	5.1	21.5
Children between 20 - 30 kg	2.5	14	8.4	17.5	6.1	23.0
Children and small adults over 30 kg	3	20	10.0	22.0	7.6	25.5
Normal and large adults	4	30	10.0	22.0	7.6	25.5
Large adults	5	40	11.5	23.5	8.7	28.5

Laryngeal Mask Airways - Indications and Contraindications

Indications:

An alternative to the face mask for achieving and maintaining control of the airway during routine anesthetic procedures.

Best suited for use in elective surgical procedures where face masks are currently used or tracheal intubation is not necessary.

Not indicated for use as a replacement for the endotracheal tube, and should be limited to use during anesthesia.

Contraindications:

The LMA does not protect against regurgitation and aspiration. It should not be used in patients with hiatal hernia (GE reflux) or suspected gastric contents. Situations where gastric contents may be present include, but are not limited to, gross or morbid obesity, pregnancy, multiple or massive injury, acute abdominal or thoracic injury, and abdominal condition associated with delayed gastric emptying or use of opiate medication prior to fasting.

Not for use in patients who have not fasted, including patients in whom fasting cannot be confirmed, and in other situations where there may be retained gastric contents.

Not for use in patients with fixed decreased pulmonary compliance, such as patients with pulmonary fibrosis.

Not for use in adult patients who are unable to understand instruction, or cannot adequately answer questions regarding their medical history.

Guidelines for Insertion of the LMA After Induction of Anesthesia

- Deflate cuff while pressing bowl of the LMA against a clean, flat surface.
- Lubricate rear (convex) surface of the LMA with water-based lubricant.
- Induce adequate depth of anesthesia (e.g., propofol 2 - 2.5 mg/kg).
- Push on back of patient's head to extend the head and flex the neck.
- Insert the LMA into patient's mouth, pressing back against the palate.
- LMA should be seen to flatten out against the palate.
- Push the LMA into oral cavity, while continuing to press against roof of mouth.
- Once past the tongue, the LMA will move easily into position.
- Stop insertion when resistance is met (LMA is at the esophageal sphincter).
- If insertion fails, consider deepening anesthetic or partially inflating LMA cuff.
- Inflate cuff (the LMA will protrude slightly).
- Connect breathing circuit, insert (soft) bite block, and secure with tape.

Reproduced with permission from reference 37.

Indications for Separation of the Two Lungs (Double-Lumen Tube Intubation) and/or One-Lung Ventilation

I. Absolute

1. Isolation of one lung from the other to avoid spillage or contamination
   A. Infection
   B. Massive hemorrhage (e.g., pulmonary artery rupture)
2. Control of the distribution of ventilation
   A. Bronchopleural fistula
   B. Bronchopleural cutaneous fistula
   C. Surgical opening of a major conducting airway
   D. Giant unilateral lung cyst or bulla
   E. Tracheobronchial-tree disruption
   F. Life-threatening hypoxemia due to unilateral lung disease
3. Unilateral bronchopulmonary lavage
   A. Pulmonary alveolar proteinosis

II. Relative

1. Surgical exposure-high priority
   A. Thoracic aortic aneurysm
   B. Pneumonectomy
   C. Thoracoscopy
   D. Upper lobectomy
   E. Mediastinal exposure
2. Surgical exposure-medium (lower) priority
   A. Middle and lower lobectomies and subsegmental resections
   B. Esophageal resection
   C. Procedures on the thoracic spine
3. Post cardiopulmonary bypass pulmonary edema/ hemorrhage after removal of totally occluding unilateral chronic pulmonary emboli
4. Severe hypoxemia due to unilateral lung disease

Reproduced with permission from reference 37.

Lung Segments

Right side	**Left side**
Upper lobe	Upper lobe
Apical	Apical-posterior
Posterior	Anterior
Anterior	
Middle lobe	Lingula
Lateral	Superior
Medial	Inferior
Lower lobe	Lower lobe
Superior	Superior
Medial basal	Anterior basal
Anterior basal	Lateral basal
Lateral basal	Posterior basal
Posterior basal	

Physiology / Pathophysiology

Cardiovascular System

Intravascular Pressure Waveforms at Various Segments of the Vascular System

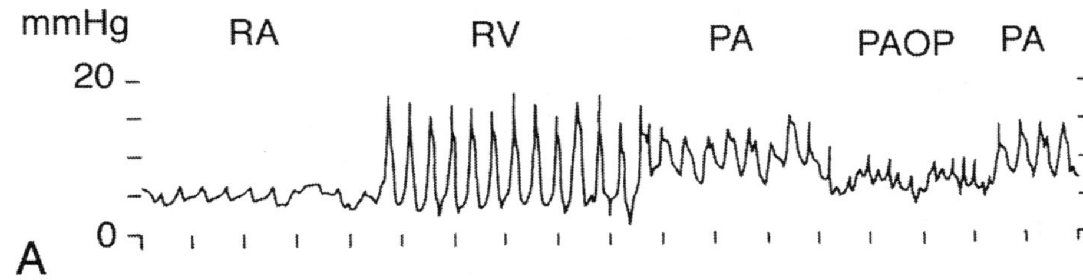

Pressure tracings and chamber locations during PA catheterization are shown. (**A**) An entire PA catheterization is shown. Specific chamber location and representative tracings are shown for the right atrium (RA) (**B**), right ventricle (RV) (**C**), pulmonary artery (PA) (**D**) and pulmonary artery occlusion pressure (PAOP) (**E**).

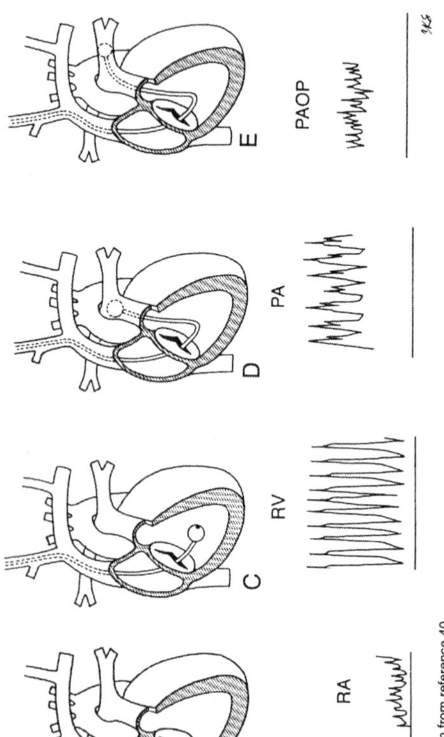

Adapted with permission from reference 40.

Normal Oxygen Saturations and Intracardiac Pressures

Location	Oxygen Saturation (%)	Intracardiac Pressure (mmHg)		
		Neonate	Child	Adult
Right atrium	75 ± 5	0 - 5	2 - 6	4 - 8
Right ventricle	75 ± 5	60/0 - 5	20/5	12 - 30/0 - 8
Pulmonary artery	75 ± 5	60/30	20/12	12 - 30/5 - 15
Left atrium	95 ± 1	4 - 5	5 - 10	0 - 12
Left ventricle	95 ± 1	70/0 - 5	90 - 110/7 - 9	90 - 140/5 -12
Aorta	95 ± 1	70/45	90 - 110/65 - 75	90 - 140/60 - 90

Hemodynamic Calculations

	Normal Range
Stroke Volume	
SV (in ml) = CO x 1000/HR	60 - 70
SVI (in ml/m^2) = SV/BSA	41 - 51
Systemic Vascular Resistance	
SVR (in dynes-sec/cm^5) = 79.96 x (ABPm-CVP)/CO	770 - 1500
SVRI (in dynes-sec/cm^5-m^2) = SVR x BSA	1970 - 2390
Pulmonary Vascular Resistance	
PVR (in dynes-sec/cm^5) = 79.96 x (PAPm-PAWP)/CO	100 - 250
PVRI (in dynes-sec/cm^5-m^2) = PVR x BSA	225 - 315
Left Cardiac Work	
LCW (in kg-m) = CO x ABPm x 0.0136	
LCWI (in kg-m/m^2) = LCW/BSA	3.4 - 4.2
Left Ventricular Stroke Work	
LVSW (in gm-m) = SV x ABPm x 0.0136	
or LVSW (in gm-m) = SV x (ABPm - PAWP) x 0.0136	
LVSWI (in gm-m/m2) = LVSW/BSA	50 - 62
Right Cardiac Work	
RCW (in kg-m) = CO x PAPm x 0.0136	
RCWI (in kg-m/m^2) = RCW/BSA	0.54 - 0.66
Right Ventricular Stroke Work	
RVSW (in gm-m) = SV x PAPm x 0.0136	
RVSWI (in gm-m/m^2) = RVSW/BSA	7.9 - 9.7

Oxygenation Calculations

	Normal Range
Arterial Oxygen Content	
CaO_2 (in ml/dl) = (1.34 x Hgb x SaO_2/100) + (PaO_2 x 0.0031)	17 - 20
Venous Oxygen Content	
CvO_2 (in ml/dl) = (1.34 x Hgb x SvO_2/100) + (PaO_2 x 0.0031)	12 - 15
Arteriovenous Oxygen Difference	
$avDO_2$ (in ml/dl) = CaO_2 - CvO_2	4.2 - 5.0
Oxygen Availability	
O_2AV (in ml/min) = CaO_2 x CO x 10	950 - 1150
O_2AVI (in ml/min) = O_2AV/BSA	50 - 650
Oxygen Consumption	
VO_2 (in ml/min) = $avDO_2$ x CO x 10	195 - 285
VO_2I (in ml/min/m^2) = VO_2/BSA	115 - 165
Oxygen Extraction Ration	
O_2ER = (CaO_2 - CvO_2)/CaO_2	0.24 - 0.28
Alveolar-Arterial Oxygen Difference	10 - 15 (on room air) or
$AaDO_2$ (in mmHg) = PAO_2 - PaO_2	10 - 65 (on 100% O_2)
where PAO_2 = FiO_2 x (PB - 47) - ($PaCO_2$ x (FiO_2 + (1 - FiO_2/RQ)	
or alternatively PAO_2 = FiO_2 x (PB - 47) - PaO_2 when RQ is assumed to be 1.	
Percent Arteriovenous Shunt	
$Qs/Qt = 100 \times \frac{Hgb \times 1.34 \times (1 - (SaO_2/100) + 0.0031(PAO_2 - PaO_2)}{Hgb \times 1.34 \times (1 - (SvO_2/100) + 0.0031(PAO_2 - PvO_2)}$	nl = 3 - 5

Adapted with permission from reference 41.

Comparison of Hemodynamic Variables

	Pediatric	Adult
Blood Volume		
Neonates	85 ml/kg	65 ml/kg
Infants	80 ml/kg	
Toddlers	80 ml/kg	
Preschoolers	75 ml/kg	
Heart Rate		
Infants	120 - 160	50 - 80
Toddlers	90 - 140	
Preschoolers	80 - 110	
School age	75 - 100	
Adolescents	60 - 90	
Systemic Arterial Pressure		
Neonates	60 - 90/20 - 60	90 - 140/60 - 90
Infants	74 - 100/50 - 70	
Toddlers	80 - 112/50 - 80	
Preschoolers	82 - 100/50 - 78	
School age	84 - 120/54 - 80	
Adolescents	94 - 140/62 - 80	
Stroke Volume		
Neonates	5 ml/beat	50 - 120 ml/beat
Preschoolers	15 ml/beat	
School age	35 ml/beat	

	Pediatric	Adult
Cardiac Index	3.5 - 4 l/min/m2	2.5 - 4 l/min/m2
SVR	800 - 1600	
PVR	80 - 240	
RA Pressure	3 mmHg	5 mmHg
RV Pressure	30/3 mmHg	25/4 mmHg
PAP	30/10 mmHg	25/12 mmHg
PCWP/LAP	8 mmHg	10 mmHg
LV Pressure	100/6 mmHg	120/10 mmHg
Aortic Pressure	100/6 mmHg	120/80 mmHg
Hemoglobin		
Neonates	17 g/dl	14 g/dl
Infants	11 g/dl	
Toddlers	12 g/dl	
Preschoolers	12.5 g/dl	
Oxygen Consumption		
Neonates	6 ml/kg/min	3 ml/kg/min
Infants	5 ml/kg/min	
Toddlers	5 ml/kg/min	
Preschoolers	6 ml/kg/min	

Adapted with permission from reference 42.

Hemodynamic Parameters in Common Clinical Situations

	RA	RV	PA	PAWP	SAP	CI	SVRI	PVRI
Normal	4 - 8 mean	12 - 30 sys / 0 - 8 dias	12 - 30 sys / 5-15 dias	0 - 12 mean	80 - 120 / 40 - 90	2.5 - 4.0	800 - 1500	150 - 240
Hypovolemic shock	↓	↓	↓	↓	↓	↓	↑	±↓
Cardiogenic shock	±↑	↑	↑	↑	↓	↓	↑	±↓
Septic shock								
Early	±↓	±↓	±↓	±↓	±↓	↑	↓	↓
Late	±N	±N	±N	±N	±N	↓	±	↑
Pulmonary embolism	↑	↑	↑	±N	±↓	↓	↑	↑
Cardiac tamponade	↑	↑ dias	±N	↑	↓	↓	↑	±↓
Cor pulmonale	↑	↑	↑	±N	±N	±↓	±↑	↑
Primary pulmonary hypertension	±N	↑	↑	±N	±N	↓	↑	↑

RA, right atrium; RV, right ventricle; PA, pulmonary artery; PAWP, pulmonary artery wedge pressure; SAP, systemic arterial pressure; CI, cardiac index; SVRI, systemic vascular resistance index; PVRI, pulmonary vascular resistance.

Reproduced with permission from reference 43.

Anesthetic Management of Valvular Heart Disease

	LV Preload	Heart Rate	Contractile State	Systemic Vascular Resistance	Pulmonary Vascular Resistance
Aortic Stenosis	↑	↓ (sinus)	Maintain	↑	Maintain
Aortic Regurgitation	↑	↑	Maintain	↓	Maintain
Mitral Stenosis	↑	↓	Maintain	Maintain	↓
Mitral Regurgitation	↑, ↓	↑, Maintain	Maintain	↓	↓
Tricuspid Stenosis	↑	↓, Maintain	Maintain	↑	Maintain
Tricuspid Regurgitation	↑	↑, Maintain	Maintain	Maintain	↓
Pulmonic Stenosis	↑	↑, ↓	Maintain	↓, Maintain	Maintain
Aortic Stenosis and Mitral Stenosis	↑	↓	Maintain	↑	↓
Aortic Stenosis and Mitral Regurgitation	↑	Maintain	Maintain	Maintain	↓
Aortic Stenosis and Mitral Regurgitation	↑	Maintain	Maintain	Maintain	Maintain
Aortic Regurgitation and Mitral Regurgitation	↑	↑	Maintain	↓	Maintain
Mitral Stenosis and Mitral Regurgitation	↑	Maintain	Maintain	↓, Maintain	↓

Adapted from reference 44.

Features of Cyanotic Congenital Heart Disease

Lesion	Anatomy	History	Physical Findings	ECG
Tetralogy of Fallot	VSD Right ventricular hypertrophy Pulmonic stenosis/atresia Overriding aorta	Cyanosis Clubbing Growth retardation	Systolic ejection murmur at LSB Systolic thrill at LSB Absent pulmonic component of S2	Right axis deviation Right ventricular hypertrophy
Transposition of great vessels	Systemic venous return to RA => RV => aorta Pulmonary venous return to LA =>LV =>pulmonary artery	Cyanosis Dyspnea Developmental delay Frequent URI	Left parasternal prominence Enlarged anterior ventricle	Right axis deviation Right ventricular hypertrophy
Tricuspid atresia	Absent tricuspid valve RV hypoplastic Retarded growth Often ASD/VSD/PDA present	Cyanosis Dyspnea Hepatomegaly Clubbing Fatigue	Single S1 Systolic murmur P pulmonale Presystolic liver pulsation Giant "A" waves on CVP	↑ LV voltage Left axis deviation
Total anomalous pulmonary venous drainage	Supracardiac connection (left or right IVC) Cardiac connection (coronary sinus or RA) Intracardiac (portal vein or IVC)	Cyanosis Heart failure Exercise intolerance	Hyperkinetic RV Widely split S2 Systolic ejection murmur	RV dominance
Hypoplastic left heart syndrome	Hypoplastic aortic arch Mitral/aortic valve atresia LV atresia and/or hypoplasia	Cyanosis Tachypnea ↓ Systemic perfusion as ductus closes	Dominant RV impulse Nonspecific systolic murmur Diminished peripheral pulses	RA enlargement RVH

Abbreviations: ASD, atrial septal defect; CVP, central venous pressure; ECG, electrocardiography; IVC, inferior vena cava; LA, left atrium; LSB, left sternal border; LV, left ventricle; LVEF, left ventricular ejection fraction; PA, pulmonary artery; PDA, patent ductus arteriosus; P, P wave; PVR, pulmonary vascular resistance; RA, right atrium; RV, right ventricle; RVEF, right ventricular ejection fraction; RVOT, right ventricular outflow tract; SVC, superior vena cava; SVR, systemic vascular resistance; URI, upper respiratory infections; VSD, ventricular septal defect.

Features of Acyanotic Congenital Heart Disease

Lesion	Anatomy	History	Physical Findings	ECG
Atrial septal defect	Ostium primum Ostium secundum Sinus venosus	Fatigue Dyspnea Arrhythmias/heart failure (4th - 5th decade of life)	Fixed splitting S2 Systolic murmur LSB Hyperdynamic RV lift	rsR' pattern over right precordium
Ventricular septal defect	Membranous Muscular	Frequent URI ↓ Growth	Systolic thrill LSB Holosystolic murmur	Rightward QRS Biventricular hypertrophy
Patent ductus arteriosus	Small, moderate, or large duct between aorta and pulmonary artery	Asymptomatic or heart failure Respiratory distress	Systolic thrill at sternal notch Continuous machinery murmur at LSB	Left atrial hypertrophy Left ventricular hypertrophy
Coarctation of aorta	Preductal Juxtaductal Postductal	Dyspnea Feeding problems Decreased growth Lower extremity claudication in older children	Gradient between upper extremity and lower extremity blood pressures	Left ventricular hypertrophy Nonspecific ST-T wave changes
Pulmonic stenosis	Valvular Infundibular Peripheral	Dyspnea Exercise intolerance Respiratory infections	Systolic ejection murmur at LSB Widely split S2	RVH Tall, peaked P waves in II
Aortic stenosis	Valvular Subvalvular Supravalvular	Dyspnea Syncope Chest pain Heart failure	Systolic ejection murmur right second ICS LV lift and/or thrill	LVH/strain

Abbreviations: CFD, color flow doppler; ECG electrocardiography; ICS, intercostal space; L => R, left to right; LSB, left sternal border; LV, left ventricle; LVEDD, left ventricular end-diastolic dimensions; LVH, left ventricular hypertrophy; PA, pulmonary artery; PVR, pulmonary vascular resistance; RA, right atrium; R => L, right to left; RV, right ventricle; RVH, right ventricular hypertrophy; 2D, two-dimensional; URI, upper respiratory infections; Vcf, velocity circumferential fiber.

Lesion	Echocardiography	Chest Radiograph	Catheterization	Pathophysiology
Tetralogy of Fallot	Subaortic VSD Anterior deviation of infundibular septum	"Boot-shaped" heart with concave PA segment and dominant RV	↑ RV pressure Gradient across RVOT Normal PA pressures Step-up in oxygen saturation at ventricular level	RVOT obstruction Left-to-right shunting ("pink" Tetralogy of Fallot) ↓ Pulmonary blood flow
Transposition of great vessels	RV to aorta and LV to PA connection	Egg-shaped enlarged heart due to RA enlargement and dominant RV	Communication between between venous ventricle and aorta Oxygen saturations reveal left-to-right shunts through ductus, atrial, or ventricular septa	Pulmonary blood flow determined by PVR; systemic oxygenation determined by intracardiac/ extracardiac mixing and pulmonary blood flow
Tricuspid atresia	Absence of tricuspid valve ↓ RV size	No pathognomonic features	↑ PA pressure ↓ PA oxygen saturation RV inaccessible with catheter	Absent RV inflow
Total anomalous pulmonary venous drainage	Normal RVEF ↑ RV EDV ↓ LVEF	Figure-of-8 or "snowman" of right and left SVC and heart	↑ RA pressure ↑ RV pressure ↑ PVR ↓ LVEF	Decreased arterial saturation coupled with pulmonary arterial or venous hypertension
Hypoplastic left heart syndrome	Aortic atresia Hypoplastic ascending aorta Mitral atresia Small or absent LV Primum ASD	Moderate cardiomegaly Increased pulmonary vascularity R heart enlargement	Confirms echocardiography findings	Flow to head and upper body via ductus arteriosus (retrograde) Flow to lower body via descending aorta (antegrade) Flow distribution between pulmonary and systemic circulations depends on PVR/SVR ratio

Reproduced with permission from reference 45.

Features of Acyanotic Congenital Heart Disease

Lesion	Anatomy	History	Physical Findings	ECG
Atrial septal defect	Ostium primum Ostium secundum Sinus venosus	Fatigue Dyspnea Arrhythmias/heart failure (4th - 5th decade of life)	Fixed splitting S2 Systolic murmur LSB Hyperdynamic RV lift	rsR' pattern over right precordium
Ventricular septal defect	Membranous Muscular	Frequent URI ↓ Growth	Systolic thrill LSB Holosystolic murmur	Rightward QRS Biventricular hypertrophy
Patent ductus arteriosus	Small, moderate, or large duct between aorta and pulmonary artery	Asymptomatic or heart failure Respiratory distress	Systolic thrill at sternal notch Continuous machinery murmur at LSB	Left atrial hypertrophy Left ventricular hypertrophy
Coarctation of aorta	Preductal Juxtaductal Postductal	Dyspnea Feeding problems Decreased growth Lower extremity claudication in older children	Gradient between upper extremity and lower extremity blood pressures	Left ventricular hypertrophy Nonspecific ST-T wave changes
Pulmonic stenosis	Valvular Infundibular Peripheral	Dyspnea Exercise intolerance Respiratory infections	Systolic ejection murmur at LSB Widely split S2	RVH Tall, peaked P waves in II
Aortic stenosis	Valvular Subvalvular Supravalvular	Dyspnea Syncope Chest pain Heart failure	Systolic ejection murmur right second ICS LV lift and/or thrill	LVH/strain

Abbreviations: CFD, color flow doppler; ECG electrocardiography; ICS, intercostal space; L => R, left to right; LSB, left sternal border; LV, left ventricle; LVEDD, left ventricular end-diastolic dimensions; LVH, left ventricular hypertrophy; PA, pulmonary artery; PVR, pulmonary vascular resistance; RA, right atrium; R => L, right to left; RV, right ventricle; RVH, right ventricular hypertrophy; 2D, two-dimensional; URI, upper respiratory infections; Vcf, velocity circumferential fiber.

Features of Acyanotic Congenital Heart Disease (continued)

Lesion	Echocardiography	Chest Radiograph	Catheterization	Pathophysiology
Atrial septal defect	↑ RA/RV size Paradoxical septal motion Septal defect on 2D, CFD, contrast echocardiography	Mild/moderate cardiac enlargement Prominent main PA	Step-up oxygen saturation at atrial level Slight ↑ RV, PA pressures	L => R shunting
Ventricular septal defect	Septal defect on 2D, CFD	↑ Pulmonary blood flow Mild/moderate cardiac enlargement	Step-up in oxygen saturation at ventricular level Normal to ≠ RV/PA pressure	L => R shunting Bidirectional shunting
Patent ductus arteriosus	Left atrial enlargement ↑ LVEDD ↑ V_{cf} shortening Ductus not usually visualized	Enlarged aorta and PA Enlarged LV	Step-up in oxygen saturation at PA Catheter passage from PA to aorta	L => R shunting (R => L shunting if PVR increased)
Coarctation of aorta	Associated anomalies such as bicuspid aortic valve seen, but coarctation not usually visualized	Left ventricular hypertrophy Notching of ribs due to to enlarged intercostal arteries	Pressure gradient across coarctation Decreased pressures in lower extremities	Upper extremity hypertension ↑ LV afterload
Pulmonic stenosis	RV hypertrophy Valvular/infundibular stenosis	Normal heart size Convex main PA Prominent RA and PV	↑ RV pressure Gradient across pulmonic valve Postobstruction pulmonary artery dilution	RV outflow obstruction
Aortic stenosis	Valvular stenosis Subvalvular membrane or hypertrophied muscle LV hypertrophy	Usually normal	↑ LV pressure Gradient between left ventricle and aorta	LV outflow obstruction

Reproduced with permission from reference 45.

Surgical Therapy for Congenital Heart Disease

Lesion	Procedure
Atrial septal defect	Suture, pericardial, prosthetic patch closure
Ventricular septal defect	Palliative - pulmonary artery banding Definitive - suture, pericardial, prosthetic patch closure
Patent ductus arteriosus	Direct ligation and division
Tetralogy of Fallot	Definitive - patch closure ventricular septal defect, pulmonary valvulotomy, right ventricular outflow track enlargement Palliative - Brock blind pulmonary valvulotomy, Blalock-Taussig subclavian-to-pulmonary artery shunt, Waterston ascending aorta-to-right pulmonary artery shunt, Potts left pulmonary artery-to-descending thoracic aorta shunt
Transposition of great vessels	Palliative - Rashkind balloon atrial septostomy Definitive - arterial switch, atrial correction (Mustard or Senning procedures), Rastelli (with ventricular septal defect)
Anomalous pulmonary venous return	Atrial patch repair
Atrioventricular canal (endocardial cushion defects)	Patch repair atrial and ventricular septal defects, mitral/tricuspid valvuloplasty
Coarctation of aorta	Subclavian flap angioplasty, resection/end-to-end anastomosis, patch angioplasty
Valvular stenosis (aortic, pulmonic, mitral)	Open valvulotomy, valve replacement
Valvular insufficiency (aortic, pulmonic, mitral)	Valvuloplasty, valve replacement
Tricuspid atresia	Balloon atrial septostomy, Fontan procedure, Glenn shunt
Pulmonic atresia	Balloon atrial septostomy, Blalock-Taussig shunt, central shunt
Hypoplastic left heart syndrome	Norwood procedure, Sade modification, transplantation

Reproduced with permission from reference 45.

Preferred Choices for Central Line Placement According to Medical Indication

Indication	First choice	Second choice	Third choice
Emergency airway management or CPR	FV	SV	AV
Brain-injured or increased intracranial pressure	FV	SV	--
Long-term parenteral nutrition	AV* or SV	IJV	--
Acute hemodialysis or plasmapheresis	SV	FV	--
Coagulopathy	FV	EJV	IJV
General access (i.e., for surgery, medicine)	IJV	FV or SV	EJV
Emergency transvenous pacemaker	RIJV	SV	LIJV or FV

*Using small silastic catheter.

AV, antecubital vein; FV, femoral vein; SV, subclavian vein; IJV, internal jugular vein; EJV, external jugular vein; R, right; L, left.

Reproduced with permission from reference 43.

Treatment of Hyperkalemia

Therapy	Dose	Onset	Duration	Complications/Limitations
Membrane Stabilization				
Calcium Gluconate or Calcium Chloride	10 - 20 ml IV 10% solution	Immediate	~1 hr	Hypercalcemia Digitalis glycosides
Redistribution				
Sodium Bicarbonate	50 - 100 mEq IV	5 to 10 min	1 to 2 hr	Alkalosis, Volume Overload
Insulin / Glucose	10 - 20 Units Regular Insulin IV/ 50 gm Glucose IV	30 min	4 - 6 hr	Hypoglycemia Hyperglycemia
Enhanced Elimination				
Loop Diuretics				
Lasix	40 mg IV	30 min	Throughout Diuresis	Volume Depletion
Bumetanide	1 mg IV			
Kayexalate	25 - 50 mg PO or PR with 70% Sorbitol	Several Hours	Hours	Patient Intolerance
Dialysis Hemodialysis Peritoneal Dialysis		Minutes	Throughout Dialysis	Dialysis

Reproduced with permission from reference 46.

Serum Potassium (K) and the ECG with Hypo- or Hyperkalemia

ECG	K ≤ 3.0 mEq/L	K > 4.0 mEq/L	K > 6.0 mEq/L	K > 8.0 mEq/L
P wave	Normal	↓ Amplitude	↓ Amplitude	Nonapparent
PR	Normal	Prolongation	Prolongation	Nonapparent
QRS	↑ Amplitude	Normal	Normal	Widening
T wave	Flat; inverted	Normal	Peaked; tented	Peaked: tented
QT	Normal	Normal	Decreased (±)	Decreased (±)
U wave	Present	Absent	Absent	Absent

Reprinted with permission from reference 7.

ECG Changes Associated with Hyperkalemia

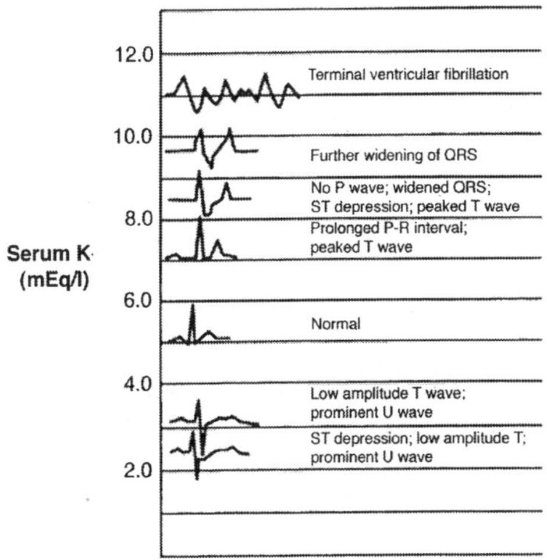

Reproduced from reference 47.

Indications for Perioperative Transesophageal Echocardiography

Category I indications: Supported by the strongest evidence or expert opinion; TEE is frequently useful in improving clinical outcomes in these settings and is often indicated, depending on individual circumstances (e.g., patient risk and practice setting).

Intraoperative evaluation of acute, persistent, and life-threatening hemodynamic disturbances in which ventricular function and its determinants are uncertain and have not responded to treatment

Intraoperative use in valve repair

Intraoperative use in congenital heart surgery for most lesions requiring cardiopulmonary bypass

Intraoperative use in repair of hypertrophic obstructive cardiomyopathy

Intraoperative use for endocarditis when preoperative testing was inadequate or extension of infection to perivalvular tissue is suspected

Preoperative use in unstable patients with suspected thoracic aortic aneurysms, dissection, or disruption who need to be evaluated quickly. Intraoperative assessment of aortic valve function in repair of aortic dissections with possible aortic valve involvement

Intraoperative evaluation of pericardial window procedures

Use in intensive care unit for unstable patients with unexplained hemodynamic disturbances, suspected valve disease, or thromboembolic problems (if other tests or monitoring techniques have not confirmed the diagnosis or patients are too unstable to undergo other tests)

Category II indications: Supported by weaker evidence and expert consensus; TEE may be useful in improving clinical outcomes in these settings, depending on individual circumstances, but appropriate indications are less certain.

Perioperative use in patients with increased risk of myocardial ischemia or infarction

Perioperative use in patients with increased risk of hemodynamic disturbances

Intraoperative assessment of valve replacement

Intraoperative assessment of repair of cardiac aneurysms

Intraoperative evaluation of removal of cardiac tumors

Intraoperative detection of foreign bodies

Intraoperative detection of air emboli during cardiotomy, heart transplant operations, and upright neurosurgical procedures

Intraoperative use during intracardiac thrombectomy

Intraoperative use during pulmonary embolectomy

Intraoperative use for suspected cardiac trauma

Category II indications (continued)

Preoperative assessment of patients with suspected acute thoracic aortic dissections, aneurysms, or disruption

Intraoperative use during repair of thoracic aortic dissections without suspected aortic valve involvement

Intraoperative detection of aortic atheromatous disease or other sources of aortic emboli

Intraoperative evaluation of pericardiectomy, pericardial effusions or evaluation of pericardial surgery

Intraoperative evaluation of anastomotic sites during heart and/or lung transplantation

Monitoring placement and function of assist devices

Category III indications: Little current scientific or expert support; TEE is infrequently useful in improving clinical outcomes in these settings, and appropriate indications are uncertain.

Intraoperative evaluation of myocardial perfusion, coronary artery anatomy, or graft patency

Intraoperative use during repair of cardiomyopathies other than hypertrophic obstructive cardiomyopathy

Intraoperative use for uncomplicated endocarditis during noncardiac surgery

Intraoperative monitoring for emboli during orthopedic procedures

Intraoperative assessment of repair of thoracic aortic injuries

Intraoperative use for uncomplicated pericarditis

Intraoperative evaluation of pleuropulmonary diseases

Monitoring placement of intraaortic balloon pumps, automatic implantable cardiac defibrillators, or pulmonary artery catheters

Intraoperative monitoring of cardioplegia administration

TEE = transesophageal echocardiography.

Reprinted with permission from reference 49.

Reported Incidence of Adverse Effects of Pulmonary Artery Catheterization

Complication	Reported Incidence (%)
Central Venous Access	
Arterial puncture	1.1 - 13
Bleeding at cut-down site (children)	5.3
Postoperative neuropathy	0.3 - 1.1
Pneumothorax	0.3 - 4.5
Air embolism	0.5
Catheterization	
Minor dysrhythmias*	4.7 - 68.9
Severe dysrhythmias (ventricular tachycardia or fibrillation)*	0.3-6 0.3 - 62.7
Right bundle-branch block	0.1 - 4.3
Complete heart block (in patients with prior LBBB)*	0 - 8.5
Catheter Residence	
Pulmonary artery rupture*	0.1 - 1.5
Positive catheter-tip cultures	1.4 - 34.8
Catheter-related sepsis	0.7 - 11.4
Thrombophlebitis	6.5
Venous thrombosis	0.5 - 66.7
Pulmonary infarction*	0.1 - 5.6
Mural thrombus*	28 - 61
Valvular/endocardial vegetations or endocarditis*.	2.2 - 100
Deaths (attributed to PA catheter)*	0.02 - 1.5

*Complications thought to be more common (or exclusively associated) with PA catheterization than with central venous catheterization.

Reproduced from reference 48.

Physiology / Pathophysiology

Nervous System

Normal Cerebrospinal Fluid Values

Pressure	90 - 180 mm H_2O
Specific gravity	1.003
Cells	Less than 5 per mm^3 (all mononuclear)
Glucose	20 mg/100 ml less than blood glucose concentration (typically 50 - 75 mg/100 ml)
Protein	15 - 40 mg/100 ml
Nonprotein Nitrogen	20 - 30 mg/ 100 ml
Sodium	140 - 150 mEq/ L
Chloride	120 - 130 mEq/L
pH	7.4 - 7.6
HCO_3	25 - 30 mEq/L

Aids in differentiation of CSF from local anesthetic:

1. Mix equal volumes of questioned liquid with thiopental. Local anesthetic and thiopental will form a precipitate.
2. Measure glucose content of questioned liquid. Only CSF will contain glucose.

CSF Findings in Intracranial Infections

	Pressure (mm H_2O)	Cell count (WBCs/μl)	Glucose (mg/dl)	Protein (mgldl)
Normal values	90 - 180	0 - 5 lymphs	50 - 75	15 - 40
Bacterial meningitis	200 - 300	100 - 5,000; neutrophils usually > 80%	Reduced (<40)	100 - 1,000
Brain abscess	180 - 300	10 - 200; lymphocytes predominate	Normal	70 - 400
Subdural empyema	200 - 300	10 - 2,000; usually lymphocytes predominate; PMNs dominate after surgery or if accompanying meningitis	Normal (<40 if meningitis)	50 - 500
Cerebral epidural abscess	180 - 250	10 - 300; lymphocytes predominate	Normal	50 - 200
Tuberculous meningitis	180 - 300	<500 lymphocytes	Reduced (<50) (increased if CSF block)	100 - 200
Cryptococcal meningitis	180 - 300	10 - 200 lymphocytes	Reduced (<40)	50 - 200
Viral meningitis	90 - 200	10 - 300 lymphocytes; early echovirus disease may have up to 80% PMN predominate	Normal (may be reduced in mumps)	50 - 100 50 - 100

Reprinted with permission from reference 51.

Pediatric Coma Scale

Eyes	Open spontaneously	4
	Open to speech	3
	Open to pain	2
	Not open	1
Motor	Obeys commands	6
	Localizes pain	5
	Flexion to pain	4
	Decorticate posturing	3
	Decerebrate posturing	2
	No reaction	1
Verbal	Obeys commands	5
	Says words	4
	Vocalizes	3
	Cries	2
	No sounds	1
"Normal" score for age:	0 - 6 mo	9
	6 - 12 mo	11
	1 - 2 yr	12
	2 - 5 yr	13
	>5 yr	14

Reprinted with permission from reference 52.

The Glasgow Coma Score

Eye Opening:		Verbal Response:		Motor Response:	
Spontaneous	4	Oriented	5	Obeys Commands	6
To Voice	3	Confused	4	Localizes To Pain	5
To Pain	2	Inappropriate Words	3	Withdraws From Pain	4
None	1	Incomprehensible Sounds	2	Flexion Posturing (Decorticate) From Pain	3
		None	1	Extension Posturing (Decerebrate) From Pain	2
				None	1

EEG Frequency Ranges

Rhythm	Associated states
Delta rhythm (0 - 3 Hz)	Deep sleep, deep anesthesia, or pathologic states (e.g., brain tumors, hypoxia, metabolic encephalopathy)
Theta rhythm (4 - 7 Hz)	Sleep and anesthesia in adults; hyperventilation in awake children and young adults
Alpha rhythm (8 - 13 Hz)	Resting, awake adult with eyes closed, predominantly seen in occipital leads
Beta rhythm (>13 Hz)	Mental activity, light anesthesia

Reprinted with permission from reference 50.

EEG Changes Associated with Anesthetic Drugs, PaO_2, $PaCO_2$ and Temperature

Increased Frequency

Barbiturates (low dose)
Benzodiazepines (low dose)
Etomidate (low dose)
N_2O (30 - 70%)
Inhalation agents (<1 MAC)
Ketamine
Hypoxia (initially)
Hypercarbia (mild)
Seizures

Decreased Frequency/Increased Amplitude

Barbiturates (moderate dose}
Etomidate (moderate dose)
Opioids
Inhalation agents (>1 MAC)
Hypoxia (mild)
Hypocarbia (moderate to extreme)
Hypothermia

Decreased Frequency/Decreased Amplitude

Barbiturates (high dose)
Hypoxia (mild)
Hypercarbia (severe)
Hypothermia (<35°C)

Electrical Silence

Barbiturates (coma dose)
Etomidate (high dose)
Isoflurane (2 MAC)
Hypoxia (severe)
Hypothermia (<15 - 20°C)
Brain death

Reprinted with permission from reference 50.

Signs and Symptoms of Intracranial Hypertension

Acute Intracranial Hypertension	Chronic Intracranial Hypertension
Physical appearance	
Bulging fontanel	Increased head circumference and compensatory skull growth
Sunset eyes	
Small, irregular pupil, dilated pupil, abnormal papillary reflexes	May have papillary abnormalities
Decreased level of consciousness, leading to abnormal posturing, seizures, altered respiratory pattern, Cushing response, brain herniation and death	May have normal mentation, mental retardation, or seizure disorder
Episodic feeding disorders or behavioral changes	
Nausea, headache, vomiting	May have nausea, headache or vomiting
Radiographic	
Dilated ventricles	Dilated ventricles
Flattening of quadrigeminal plate cistern; flattening the posterior 3rd ventricle (ascending transtentorial herniation)	"Copper beaten" skull

Reprinted with permission from reference 53.

Effects of Anesthetics on CBF/$CMRO_2$

Anesthetic	CBF	$CMRO_2$	Coupling	Vasodilatation
Halothane	↑↑↑	↓	No	Yes
Enflurane	↑↑	↓	No	Yes
Isoflurane	↑ or 0	↓↓	Yes	Yes
N_2O alone	↑	↑	Probably yes	Not known
N_2O with volatile anesthetics	↑	↑	Probably yes	
N_2O with intravenous anesthetics	0	0	-	-
Thiopental	↓↓↓	↓↓↓	Yes	No
Etomidate	↓↓↓	↓↓↓	Yes	No
Propofol	↓↓	↓↓	Yes	No
Midazolam	↓↓	↓↓	Yes	No
Ketamine	↑↑	↑	Yes	Yes
Fentanyl	↓ or 0	↓ or 0	-	No
Sufentanil	Not known	0		
Alfentanil	Not known	Not known	-	

0= no change; - = data inconclusive or no data

Reprinted with permission from reference 50.

Avoid N_2O

Effects of Intravenous and Inhaled Agents on Sensory Evoked Potentials

	BAEPs		cSSEPs		VEPs	
	Latency	Amplitude	Latency	Amplitude	Latency	Amplitude
Intravenous Agents						
Thiopental						
4 - 6 mg/kg	0	0	0	0	-	-
20 mg/kg	↑	0	↑	↓	↑	↓
75 mg/kg	↑	↓	↑	↓	↑	↓
Pentobarbital						
9 - 18 mg/kg	↑	↓	↑	↓	↑	↓
Droperidol						
0.1 mg/kg	-	-	↑	↓	-	-
Diazepam						
0.1 mg/kg	0	0	↑	↓	-	-
Midazolam	-	-	0	↓	-	-
Meperidine	-	-	↑	↑/↓	-	-
Morphine	-	-	↑	↓	-	-
Fentanyl	0	0	↑	↓	-	-
Sufentanil	0	0	0	↓	-	-

	BAEPs		cSSEPs		VEPs	
	Latency	Amplitude	Latency	Amplitude	Latency	Amplitude
Intravenous Agents						
Alfentanil	0	0	0	↓	-	-
Etomidate 0.05 - 0.3 mg/kg/min	0	0	↑	↑	-	-
Propofol 2 - 6 mg/kg	0	0	↑	↓	-	-
Inhalation Agents						
Enflurane	↑	0	↑	↑*	↑	↓
Halothane	↑	0	↑	↓	↑	0
Isoflurane	↑	0	↑	↓*	↑	↓
Nitrous oxide	0	0	0	↓	↑	↓

BAEPs = brain stem auditory evoked potentials, cSSEPs = cortical somatosensory evoked potentials, VEPs = visual evoked potentials, ↑ = increased, ↓ = decreased, 0 = no change, - = no data.

* 1.5 MAC enflurane and isoflurane (but not halothane) will occasionally abolish the cortical evoked response to median nerve stimulation.

Reprinted with permission from reference 50.

Reflexes and Corresponding Innervation

Reflex	Nerve Root	Peripheral Nerve
Biceps	C5,6	Musculocutaneous nerve
Brachioradialis	C5,6	Radial Nerve
Triceps	C7,8	Radial Nerve
Superficial Abdominal Reflexes		
Upper abdomen	T8,9,10	
Lower abdomen	T11,12	
Cremasteric	L1,2	
Anal	S3,4	
Quadriceps	L3,4	Femoral Nerve
Hamstrings, Medial	L5	Sciatic Nerve
Hamstring, Lateral	S1	Sciatic Nerve
Gastrocnemius-soleus	S1,2	Tibial Nerve

Clinical, Pathophysiologic, and Monitoring Thresholds in Cerebral Ischemia

CBF (ml/100 g/min)	Clinical Changes	Pathophysiologic Changes	Monitored
50	Normal		
23	Reversible paralysis		EEG slowing, EP change
20		Na^+-K^+ pump dysfunction	
18	Infarction		EEG flat
15			EP absent
10		K^+ efflux, Ca^{2+} influx	

Reprinted with permission from reference 54.

Glossary of Neurologic Monitor Characteristics

Term	Definition
Bias	Average difference (positive or negative) between monitored values and "gold standard" values
Precision	Standard deviation of the differences (bias) between the measurements
Sensitivity	Probability that the monitor will demonstrate cerebral ischemia when cerebral ischemia is present
Positive predictive value	Probability that cerebral ischemia is present when the monitor suggests cerebral ischemia
Specificity	Probability that the monitor will not demonstrate cerebral ischemia when cerebral ischemia is not present
Negative predictive value	Probability that cerebral ischemia is not present when the monitor reflects no cerebral ischemia
Threshold value	The value used to separate acceptable (i.e., no ischemia present) from unacceptable (i.e., ischemia present)
Speed	The time elapsed from the onset of actual ischemia or the risk of ischemia until the monitor provides evidence

Reprinted with permission from reference 54.

Techniques for Assessing Cerebral Circulation

Characteristic	Evoked Potentials	EEG	CBF (^{133}Xe Clearance)	CBF (Transcranial Doppler Flow Velocity)	ICP Monitoring	Brain Metabolic Monitoring (Jugular Venous Saturation)	Brain Metabolic Monitoring (Near-Infrared Spectroscopy)
Bias	NA	NA	± 5%	NA	Excellent	Gold standard	Not established
Precision	NA	NA	± 5%	NA	Excellent	Gold standard	Not established
Sensitivity	High for ischemia	Good for ischemia; sensitive to drug effects	Good for 5% change	Good for CBF change (relative)	Good for ICP change; poor for ischemia	Good for global; poor for regional	Good for severe global desaturation
Positive predictive value	Good for ischemia	Poor for ischemia	Good for CBF decrease	Good for CBF change	Good for ICP change; poor for ischemia	Good for global; poor for regional	Not established
Specificity	High for ischemia	Poor for ischemia	Poor for ischemia; good for CBF decrease	Good for CBF change	Good for ICP change; Poor for ischemia	Good	Not established

Characteristic	Evoked Potentials	EEG	CBF (^{133}Xe Clearance)	CBF (Transcranial Doppler Flow Velocity)	ICP Monitoring	Brain Metabolic Monitoring (Jugular Venous Saturation)	Brain Metabolic Monitoring (Near-Infrared Spectroscopy)
Negative predictive value	Good for ischemia	Fair for ischemia	Poor for ischemia	Poor for ischemia; good for vasospasm	Good for ICP change; poor for ischemia	Good	Not established
Thershold Definition	Ischemia (CBF 15 - 23 ml/100 g/min)	Ischemia (CBF 18 - 23 ml/100 g/min)	Can be set at a desired level	Interpatient variability	15 - 20 mm Hg or < 50 mm Hg cerebral perfusion pressure	Saturation < 50	Probably similar to jugular saturation
Speed	Good	Good	Poor	Poor	Good (once inserted)	Fair (good if continuous)	Excellent
Utility in clinical:							
Diagnosis	Good	Good	Poor	Good	Poor	Poor	Untested
Surveillance	Poor	Fair	Poor	Fair in SAH	Good (CHI)	Poor (good continuous)	Should be excellent
Prognosis	Good	Fair	Fair	Fari in SAH	Good (CHI)	Fair	Untested
Goal-directed therapy	Poor	Poor	Poor	Untested	Fair (CHI) Reye's syndrome	Untested	Potentially valuable, but untested

Reprinted with permission from reference 55.

Physiology / Pathophysiology

Endocrine System

Peak Action and Duration of Hypoglycemic Agents

Agent	Onset (hours)	Peak Action (hours)	Duration (hours)
Insulins (SQ)			
Rapid			
Regular	1	2 - 4	6 - 8
Semilente	1	2 - 6	10 - 12
Intermediate			
NPH (Neutral protamine)	2	6 - 12	18 - 24
Lente	2	6 - 12	18 - 24
Long-acting			
Protamine zinc (PZI)	4	14 - 24	36
Ultralente	4	16 - 24	36

	Onset (hours)	Duration (hours)
Sulfonylureas		
Tolbutamide (Orinase)	1	8 - 12
Glipizide (Glucotrol)	1	8 - 24
Acetohexamide (Tolinase)	4 - 6	12 - 16
Glyburide (Diabeta)	1 - 4	18 - 24
Chlorpropamide (Diabinese)	1 - 4	24 - 72

Pediatric Endocrine Levels: Normal Values[a]

Pituitary Gland

Growth hormone	Basal	Low-undetectable
	After stimulation	>15 mU/L
ACTH	Basal (0900 hours)	20 - 80 ng/L
TSH	Basal	<5 mU/L
	After TRH	5 - 25 mU/L
LH	Basal	
	Prepubertal	0.6 - 1.7 U/L
	Pubertal	0.8 - 8.7 U/L
	After LHRH	
	Prepubertal	1.5 - 11.9 U/L
	Pubertal	5.9 - 48.8 U/L
FSH	Basal	
	Prepubertal	0.6 - 3.4 U/L
	Pubertal	0.6 - 4.9 U/L
	After LHRH	
	Prepubertal	3.9 - 5.6 U/L
	Pubertal	2.2 - 8.0 U/L
ADH	Basal	1 - 5 pmol/L
	Plasma osmolarity	275 - 295 mOsm/L

Thyroid Gland

Total T_4	55 - 150 nmol/L (4 - 12 µg/dl)
Total T_3	1.2 - 3.1 nmol/L (78 - 200 ng/dl)
TSH	<5 mU/L
TBG	12 - 31 ng/L

Parathyroid Glands

PTH	<1.0 ng/ml
Calcitonin	<0.08 ng/L
Serum calcium	2.26 - 2.80 mmol/L (9 - 11 mg/dl)
Serum phosphate	0.8 - 1.45 mmol/L (2.5 - 4.5 mg/dl)
Serum magnesium	0.7 - 1.2 mmol/L (1.7 - 2.9 mg/dl)

Adrenal Cortex

Cortisol	140 - 800 nmol/L (5 - 29 µg/dl)
17-OHP	<15 nmol/L (<45 ng/dl)
11-Deoxycortisol	<60 nmol/L

Adrenal Medulla

Urinary excretion of catecholamines and metabolites varies with age, and also shows a diurnal variation. It is usual to take a 24-hour collection for assessment.

Normal ranges for children:

VMA	<35 µmol/d
Metadrenaline	<6.5 µmol/d

Pediatric Endocrine Levels: Normal Values (continued)

Pancreas

Plasma insulin	<10 mU/L
Plasma glucose (fasting)	2.8 - 6.5 mmol/L (50 - 117 mg/dl)
Hemoglobin $A1_c$	5.7 - 8.0%

[a]These values are a guide only - results may vary depending upon individual laboratory standards and techniques.

Reprinted with permission from reference 56.

Replacement Therapy for Pediatric Patients

Drug	Dose
Hydrocortisone	10 - 25 mg/m^2/d PO in 3 divided doses
Prednisone	4 - 5 mg/m^2/d PO in 2 divided doses
Desmopressin (DDAVP)	2.5 - 15µg/kg every 12 hours intranasally
DOCA	1.0 mg/d IM
Fludrocortisone	0.05 - 0.1 mg/d PO
Levothyroxine sodium (Synthroid)	Infants: 6 - 10 µg/kg/d PO 1 - 5 years: 5 - 6 µg/kg/d 6 - 12 years: 4 - 5 µg/kg/d >12 years: 2 - 3 µg/kg/d
Vasopressin (Pitressin)	2.5 - 5 U, 2 - 4 times daily IM or SC

Reprinted with permission from reference 56.

Multi-Donor Transplantation: Donor Management

Hormone Replacement for Donors Exhibiting Endocrine Dysfunction

	Dose
Tri-iodothyronine	Bolus: 4 µg Infusion: 3 µg/hr
ADH (Vasopressin)	Bolus: 1 U Infusion: 1.5 U/hr
Insulin	Infusion to maintain normal blood sugar (minimum 1 U/hr)
Epinephrine	Infusion 0 - 0.5 µg/kg/hr, depending on afterload
Hydrocortisone	Bolus: 5 µg/kg

Reprinted with permission from reference 57.

Steroid Relative Potencies and Doses

Steroid	Relative Potency‡ Glucocorticoid	Mineralocorticoid	Equivalent Dose (mg)	Activity (hr)
Short-acting (8-12 hour duration)				
Hydrocortisone (Cortisol, Solu-Cortef)	1.0	1.0	20	8
Cortisone	0.8	0.8	25	8
Aldosterone	0.3	3000	--	--
Intermediate (12-36 hour duration)				
Prednisone	4	0.8	5	24
Pednisolone	4	0.8	5	36
Methylprednisolone (Solu-Medrol)	5	0.5	4	36
Triamcinolone	5	0	*	1 - 6 weeks
Fludrocortisone	10	125	--	--
Long-acting (>48 hour duration)				
*Dexamethasone (Decadron)	25 - 40	0	0.5	72

‡The glucocorticoid and mineralocorticoid activities refer to the antiinflammatory potency and the relative sodium retention, respectively.
*If discontinued acutely , can have a hypothalamic-pituitary-adrenal axis suppression - need to cover for up to 96 hrs.

High dose steroids for peri-operative coverage - based on length (and quantity) on steroids and length of surgical procedure. Examples:

1) 5 mg prednisone po QOD x 1 month => 5 mg po premed and then 5 - 10 mg hydrocortisone intraop.
2) 10 mg prednisone po QD x yrs => 5 - 10 mg methylprednisolone IV intraop ± po premed
3) High dose steroids (eg, Crohn's) => hydrocortisone IV 100/100/100 mg pre- , intra- , and post-op.

Steroids of choice in an asthmatic patient = Dexamethasone and Methylprednisolone
Steroids of choice in a patient with adrenal insufficiency = Hydrocortisone

Tests for Thyroid Gland Function

	T_4	RT_3R	T_3	TSH
Hyperthyroidism	Elevated	Elevated	Elevated	Normal or Low Elevated
Primary Hypothyroidism	Low	Low	Low or Normal	Elevated
Secondary Hypothyroidism	Low	Low	Low	Low
Sick Euthyroidism (decreased peripheral conversion T_4 to T_3)	Normal	Normal	Low	Normal
Pregnancy	Elevated	Low	Normal	Normal

T_4 = total serum thyroxine, RT_3U = T_3 resin uptake, T_3 = serum triiodothyronine, TSH = thyroid-stimulating hormone.

Reprinted with permission from reference 28.

Physiology / Pathophysiology

Hematologic System

Estimation of Allowable Blood Loss

$$ABL = \frac{EBV\,(Hb_{initial} - Hb_{target})}{Hb_{initial}}$$

ABL = Allowable blood loss

EBV = Estimated blood volume

$Hb_{initial}$ = Initial hemoglobin

Hb_{target} = Target hemoglobin (minimally acceptable hemoglobin)

Standard Surgical Blood Order Schedule for Elective Surgery

Procedure	Preoperative Orders
General Surgery	
Abdominal-perineal resection	2
Breast Biopsy	T&S
Cholecystectomy	T&S
Colon resection	2
Colostomy	T&S
Esophageal resection	4
Gastric tumor or ulcer resection	2
Gastrectomy	2
Gastric bypass, gastroplasty	T&S
Gastrostomy, ileostomy	T&S
Hemorrhoidectomy	T&S
Hernia, diaphragmatic	2
Hernia, hiatal	2
Hernia repair	T&S
Hepatic resection	6
Kidney transplant	4
Laparotomy	T&S
Laparoscopy	T&S
Lymphadenectomy	2
Mastectomy:	
simple	T&S
radical	2
Nissen fundoplication	T&S
Pancreatectomy	4
Parathyroidectomy	T&S
Parotidectomy	T&S
Polypectomy, transabdominal	2
Porto-caval, spleno-renal shunt	4
Renal artery graft	2
Renal transplant	2

Procedure	Preoperative Orders
General Surgery (continued)	
Splenectomy	2
Small bowel resection	2
Thyroidectomy	T&S
Vagotomy	2
Cardiopulmonary - Vascular - Thoracic	
Aneurysm, abdominal aortic	6
Aneurysm, peripheral vascular	2
Aneurysm, thoracic aortic	6
ASD repair	4
Bronchopleural fistula repair	2
Bypass graft:	
aorta femoral	6
aorta iliac	5
femoro-popliteal	2
Cardiac bypass procedure	
adults	6
children	4
Carotid endarterectomy	T&S
Coarctation of aorta, correction	2
Epicardial pacemaker implant	T&S
Lung biopsy	T&S
Mediastinal tumor resection	2
Mediastinoscopy	T&S
Mitral commissurotomy	4
Patent ductus repair	2
Pericardiectomy	2
Pleural abrasion	2
Thoracotomy:	
lobectomy	2
open lung biopsy	T&S
pneumonectomy	3
Tracheal resection	4
Valve replacement	6
Gynecology - Obstetrics	
Suction abortion	T&S
Anterior - posterior repair	T&S
Cesarean delivery	T&S
D&C, conization of cervix	T&S
Ectopic pregnancy	2
Hysterectomy:	
abdominal, vaginal	T&S
radical (Wertheim)	3
Laparoscopy	T&S
Oophorectomy	T&S
Ovarian cystectomy, wedge resection	T&S

Procedure	Preoperative Orders
Gynecology - Obstetrics (continued)	
Ovarian malignancy (debulking)	3
Pelvic exenteration, lymphadenectomy	4
Salpingo-oophorectomy	T&S
Tuboplasty	T&S
Tubal ligation	T&S
Uterine suspension	T&S
Vulvectomy, simple	T&S
Vulvectomy, radical with node dissection	4
Neurosurgery	
Cervical spondylosis (decompressive)	4
Cordotomy	T&S
Cranioplasty	2
Craniotomy:	
acute subdural, epidural hematoma	2
aneurysm clipping	3
posterior fossa	3
tumor (meningioma) resection	4
tumor (such as glioma, astrocytoma, glioblastoma, any metastatic tumor) resection	2
Laminectomy, cervical/lumbar discectomy	T&S
Lumbar fusion	3
Lumbar spondylosis (decompressive)	2
Shunt, V-P or V-A	T&S
Spinal cord tumor	4
Transsphenoidal hypophysectomy	2
Orthopedics	
Amputation, leg	T&S
Hip nailing	2
Rotator cuff repair	T&S
Shoulder repair	T&S
Spinal fusion:	3
with instrumentation	4
Tibial osteotomy	T&S
Total hip arthroplasty	4
Total hip revision	5
Total knee arthroplasty	2
Total shoulder arthroplasty	2
Otolaryngology	
Brachial cleft cyst	T&S
Caldwell-Luc procedure	T&S
Carotid body tumor resection	4
Ethmoidectomy	T&S
Glossectomy or hemiglossectomy	2
Jaw, neck, tongue dissection	4

Procedure	Preoperative Orders
Otolaryngology(continued)	
Laryngectomy:	2
with radical neck	4
Mandibulectomy or maxillectomy	2
Mastoidectomy	T&S
Radical neck dissection	2
Rhinotomy	3
Septoplasty	T&S
Tonsillectomy	T&S
Tracheostomy	T&S
Thyroglossal duct cyst resection	T&S
Plastic Surgery	
Cleft palate repair	T&S
Decubitus ulcer repair	2
Mammoplasty:	
augmentation, reduction	T&S
reconstruction	4
Urology	
Adrenalectomy	2
Bladder tumor fulguration	2
Cystectomy	2
Cystotomy	T&S
Cystectomy, radical	4
Ileal conduit	2
Nephrolithotomy	2
Nephrostomy	T&S
Nephrectomy	2
Orchiectomy	T&S
Prostatectomy:	
perineal, suprapubic	2
perineal, radical	3
transurethral resection	T&S
Pelviolithotomy	T&S
Pyelolithotomy	T&S
Pyeloplasty	T&S
Transurethral resection bladder tumor	T&S
Ureteral reimplantation and repair	T&S
Ureterolithotomy	T&S

For surgical procedures where less than 10% of patients require blood, but for which there is a potential transfusion requirement, a type and screen (T&S) with no crossmatch is appropriate.

Adapted with permission from reference 58.

Available Blood Components

Component	Content	Indications	Volume	Shelf Life
RBCs Whole	RBCs and WBCs, platelet debris, plasma, fibrinogen	Red cell volume and plasma volume replacement	450 ± 50 mL	Heparin 48 hrs ADSOL 42 days ACD 21 days CPD 28 days CPDA-I 35 days
Packed	RBCs, WBCs, some plasma, platelet debris	Red cell volume replacement	200 mL	same as whole blood
Frozen	No plasma, minimal WBCs & platelet debris	Red cell volume replacement in special circumstances	160-190 mL	Frozen: 3 years Thawed: 24 hours
Platelets	Platelets, few WBCs, some plasma	Platelet count less than 50,000-100,000, clinical signs of dilutional thrombocytopenia and/or platelet dysfunction	30-50 mL/unit	Pheresis: 24 hours Room temperature: 5 days, Frozen with DMSO: 3 years
Fresh Frozen Plasma	Plasma proteins, all coagulation factors	Bleeding from factor deficiencies, antithrombin III deficiency, massive transfusions, coumadin reversal	200-250 mL	Thawed: 6-24 hours Frozen: I year

Component	Content	Indications	Volume	Shelf Life
Cryoprecipitate	Factors VIII, XIII, fibrinogen, fibronectin, von Willebrand's Factor	Hemophilia A, von Willebrand's disease, fibrinogen deficiency	25 mL/unit	Thawed: 4-6 hours Frozen: I year
Factor VIII Concentrate	Factor VIII, fibrinogen von-Willebrand's Factor	Hemophilia A (Classic Hemophilia)	Lyophilized (requires reconstitution)	2-8°C: I year Room temp: 3 months
Factor IX Concentrates (Konyne, Proplex)	Factors II, VII, IX, X	Hemophilia B (Christmas disease)	Lyophilized (requires reconstitution)	2-8°C: I year Room temp: I month
Albumin 25%	Albumin	Volume expansion, maintenance of intravascular oncotic pressure	50 mL	3-5 years
5%	Albumin and saline		250 mL and 500 mL	3-5 years
Plasma Protein Fraction	Albumin, alpha globulin, beta globulin	Volume expansion, maintenance of intravascular oncotic pressure	250 mL	3-5 years

Reprinted with permission from reference 59.

Key Laboratory Tests in Some Common Anemias

Anemia Type	Class‡	RI	MCV	MCH	Fe/TIBC	% Fe Saturation	Other
Aplastic/Hypoplastic	Hypoproliferative	↓	N or ↑	N	N	N	Hypoplastic or aplastic marrow
Myelophthisic	Hypoproliferative	↓	N	N	Variable	Variable	BM invasion with tumor fibrosis Teardrops, NRBC in smear
Chronic inflammation	Hypoproliferative	↓	N	N or Sl ↓	↓/↓	N or Sl ↓	↑ RE iron stores ↓ Sideroblasts
Iron deficiency	Hypoproliferative + Cytoplasmic maturation defect	↓ ↓	↓	↓	↓/↑	<10%	↓ RE iron stores ↓ Sideroblasts
Megaloblastic anemias	Nuclear maturation defect	↓	↑	N	↑/↑	↑↑	Megaloblasts in BM
Hemolytic anemias (uncomplicated)	Hemolysis	↑	N or ↑*	N	Variable	Variable	May be normocytic or show characteristic abnormalities on blood smear
Uncomplicated acute blood loss	Blood loss	↑	N or ↑*	N	N	N	
Combined anemias	Variable						

‡: Pathophysiologic
*: With marked reticulocytosis.
NRBC: Nucleated red blood cells
Fe/TIBC: Iron/total iron binding capacity

N: Normal
RE: Reticulo-endothelial
MCV: Mean cell volume
MCH: Mean cell hemoglobin

BM: Bone marrow
RI: Retic Index
SI: Slight

Reproduced with permission from reference 60.

Normal Red Cell Values and Platelet Counts in Adults

Determination	Men		Women	
	Mean	95% range	Mean	95% range
Red cell count, x $10^6/\mu l$ (or x 10^{12}/liter)	5.1	4.5 - 5.9	4.6	4.1 - 5.1
Hemoglobin, g/dl	15.3	14.2 - 16.9	13.9	12.2 - 15.0
Hematocrit, l/l x 100	45.9	41.8 - 49.0	41.4	38.6 - 45.7
MCV, fl	90	83 - 99	90	83 - 99
MCH, pg	30	28 - 32	30	28 - 32
MCHC, g/dl	33	32 - 36	34	32 - 36
Reticulocytes, %	1.0	0.5 - 1.8	1.2	0.5 - 2.2
x 10^4/l	50	25 - 100	55	25 - 120
Platelet count, x 10^9/l	245	160 - 340	248	150 - 380

Reprinted with permission from reference 61.

Normal White Cell Values and Differential Counts in Adults

Determination	Mean values: Cell counts, x $10^3/\mu l$	Mean values: % of total	95% range cell counts, x $10^3/\mu l$
White cell count	7,200	100	3,900 - 10,900
Differential cell count			
Neutrophils	4,200	58	2,000 - 6,800
Band forms	200	3	100 - 800
Eosinophils	100	2	<100 - 200
Basophils	<10	<1	<10 - 20
Monocytes	300	4	100 - 800
Lymphocytes	2,400	33	1,000 - 4,200

Reprinted with permission from reference 61.

Routine Screening Tests for Evaluation of Hemostasis

Defect	Platelet Count	Bleeding Time	Prothrombin Time	Activated Partial Thromboplastin Time
Thrombocytopenia	Decreased	Prolonged	Normal	Normal
Blood Vessel Defects	Normal	Prolonged	Normal	Normal
Platelet Function Defects	Normal	Prolonged	Normal	Normal
Factor VII Deficiency	Normal	Normal	Prolonged	Normal
Factor II, V or X Deficiency	Normal	Normal	Prolonged	Prolonged
Factor VIII or IX Deficiency	Normal	Normal	Normal	Prolonged
von Willebrand's Disease	Normal	Prolonged	Normal	Prolonged
Dysfibrinogenemia	Normal	Variable	Variable	Variable
Afibrinogenemia	Normal	Variable	Prolonged	Prolonged
Factor XIII Deficiency*	Normal	Normal	Normal	Normal

*The urea clot lysis test is diagnostic

Screening Tests for Patients with Bleeding
(In the presence of a normal bleeding time)

PT	Prolonged	Prolonged	Prolonged	Normal	Normal
aPTT	Prolonged	Prolonged	Normal	Prolonged	Normal
Platelets	Decreased	Normal	Normal	Normal	Normal
Disorder	DIC Liver Disease Sepsis	Vit K Deficiency Liver Disease Heparin Coumadin Deficiency of Factors II, V, X or fibrinogen	Vit K Deficiency Liver Disease Deficiency of Factor VII Coumadin	von Willebrand's Heparin Deficiency of Factors VIII, IX or XI	von Willebrand's Deficiency of Factor XIII or α2-antiplasmin Mild platelet abnormality

Effects of Some Commonly Used Agents on Coagulation Perimeters

Agent	Bleeding Time	Prothrombin Time	Activated Thrombo-plastin Time	Activated Clotting Time	Time to Peak Effect	Time to Normal Hemostasis Post-therapy	Comments
Aspirin	↑↑↑	–	–	–	Hours	1 week	Platelet function not accurately predicted by bleeding time
Other NSAIDs	↑↑↑	–	–	–	Hours	3 - 5 days	Platelet function not accurately predicted by bleeding time
Heparin, regular							
Intravenous	↑	↑	↑↑↑	↑↑↑	Minutes	4 - 6 hours	Monitor activated clotting time or activated thromboplastin time
Subcutaneous	↑	↑	↑↑	↑↑	1 hour	4 - 6 hours	Activated thromboplastin time may remain normal; monitor anti-Xa activity
Heparin, low molecular weight							
Subcutaneous	–	–	–/↑	–/↑	12 hours	1 - 2 days	Activated thromboplastin time may remain normal; monitor anti-Xa activity
Thrombolytic agents	↑↑↑	↑	↑	–	Minutes	1 - 2 days	Frequently administered along with intravenous heparin

↑ : clinically insignificant increase; ↑↑ : possibly clinically significant increase; ↑↑↑ : clinically significant increase

Appropriateness Criteria for Use of the PT and APPT Tests

Preprocedure Evaluation

- Evidence of liver disease on physical examination prior to an invasive procedure
- History of malabsorption or malnutrition noted prior to an invasive procedure
- Clinical history unavailable prior to an invasive procedure
- Any indication listed below if noted or detected prior to an invasive procedure

Evaluation of Abnormal Bleeding

- Active bleeding or evidence of abnormal bleeding on physical examination
- History of abnormal, excessive, or spontaneous bleeding

Use of Anticoagulants

- Recent or current use of therapeutic heparin or warfarin

Evaluation of Abnormal Coagulation

- Suspected or proved thromboembolism
- Suspected or proved disseminated intravascular coagulation

Reprinted with permission from reference 62.

Analysis of the Thrombelastograph

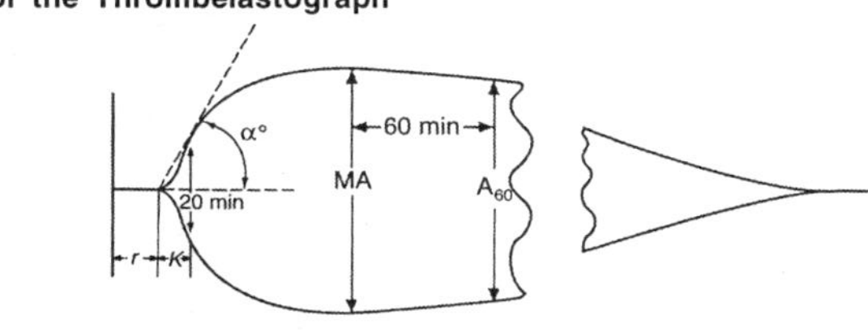

Quantification of TEG variables. *r* = Reaction time (time from sample placement in the cuvette until TEG tracing amplitude reaches 2 mm (normal range 6 - 8 min)). This represents the rate of initial fibrin formation and is related functionally to plasma clotting factor and circulating inhibitor activity (intrinsic coagulation). Prolongation of the *r* time may be a result of coagulation factor deficiencies, anticoagulation (heparin) or severe hypofibrinogenemia. A small *r* value may be present in hypercoagulability syndromes. *K* = clot formation time (normal range 3 - 6 min); measured from *r* time to the point where the amplitude of the tracing reaches 20 mm. The coagulation time represents the time taken for a fixed degree of viscoelasticity to be achieved by the forming clot, as a result of fibrin build up and cross linking. It is effected by the activity of the intrinsic clotting factors, fibrinogen and platelets. Alpha angle (α°) (normal range 50 - 60°) = angle formed by the slope of the TEG tracing from the *r* to the *K* value. It denotes speed at which solid clot forms. Decreased values may occur with hypofibrinogenemia and thrombocytopenia. Maximum amplitude (MA) (normal range 50 - 60 mm) = greatest amplitude on the TEG trace and is a reflection of the absolute strength of the fibrin clot. It is a direct function of the maximum dynamic properties of fibrin and platelets. Platelet abnormalities, whether *qualitative* or quantitative, substantially disturb the MA. A60 (normal range = MA - 5 mm) = amplitude of the tracing 60 min after MA is achieved. It is a measure of clot lysis or retraction. The clot lysis index (CLI) (normal range >85%) is derived as A60/MA X 100(%). It measures the amplitude as a function of time and reflects loss of clot integrity as a result of lysis.

Modified with permission from reference 63.

Specific Hemostatic Defects Produce Characteristic TEG Traces

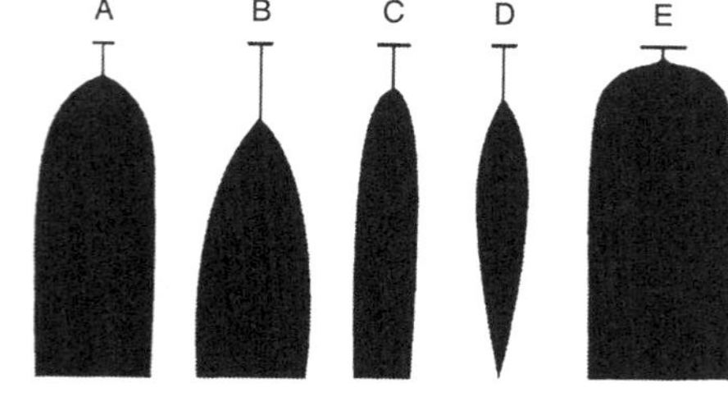

A = Normal trace.

B = Hemophilia: marked prolongation of *r* and *K* times. Decreased alpha angle.

C = Thrombocytopenia: Normal *r* and *rK* times, decreased MA (< 40 mm).

D = Fibrinolysis: CLI < 85 %.

E = Hypercoagulability: short *r* time, increased MA and steep clot formation rate.

Reprinted with permission from reference 63.

Differential Diagnosis of Bleeding

	Coagulopathies	Platelet Disorders
Positive Family History	Common	Rare
Bleeding from superficial cuts and scratches	Minimal	Persistent
Delayed Bleeding	Common	Rare
Ecchymosis	Common, often large	Common, often small and multiple
Epistaxis	Uncommon	Common
Hemarthrosis	Characteristic	Rare
Hematuria	Common	Uncommon
Petechiae/Purpura	Rare	Common

Causes of Thrombophilia

Familial Thrombophilic (Inherited) Disorders

Established association
- APC resistance
- AT-III deficiency
- Protein C deficiency (heterozygous autosomal dominant)
- Protein C deficiency (homozygous autosomal recessive)
- Protein S deficiency
- Dysfibrinogenemia*

Unestablished association
- Plasminogen deficiency
- Heparin cofactor II deficiency
- Increased histidine-rich glycoprotein
- Decreased plasminogen activator activity

Acquired Thromboembolic Disorders

Malignancy

Antiphospholipid antibody

Paroxysmal nocturnal hemoglobinuria

Myeloproliferative syndrome

Nephrotic syndrome

Estrogen therapy for infertility

Reduction in postoperative fibrinolytic activity

* Rare.

APC indicates activated protein C; AT-III, antithrombin III.

Reprinted with permission from reference 64.

Clinical Manifestations of Thrombophilia

Family history of venous thrombosis
Thrombosis at a young age
Recurrent venous thrombosis
Idiopathic venous thrombosis
Venous thrombosis following minimal provocation (eg, antepartum thrombosis, thrombosis after a long car ride or airplane flight while taking oral contraceptives)
Venous and arterial thrombosis in combination
Thrombosis in an unusual site
- Inferior vena cava
- Mesenteric vein thrombosis
- Cerebral vein thrombosis
- Renal vein thrombosis
- Hepatic vein thrombosis
- Axillary vein thrombosis

Recurrent thrombosis despite adequate anticoagulant therapy (malignant disease)

Some clinical manifestations of thrombophilia are particularly characteristic of special thrombophilic disorders. These deficiencies are shown in parentheses.

Reprinted with permission from reference 64.

Risk Factors for Venous Thromboembolism

- Age > 60 y
- Extensive surgery*
- Previous venous thromboembolism
- Marked immobility, preoperative or postoperative
- Major orthopedic surgery
  - Hip surgery
  - Major knee surgery
- Fracture of pelvis, femur, or tibia
- Surgery for malignant disease
- Postoperative sepsis
- Major medical illness
  - Heart failure
  - Inflammatory bowel disease
  - Sepsis
  - Myocardial infarction

---

* Risk of postoperative thrombosis is increased by patient's age, presence of varicose veins, obesity, and length of surgery.

Reprinted with permission from reference 64.

Risk Categories for Venous Thromboembolism

Thrombolic Event	Category 1, Low Risk	Category 2, Moderate Risk*	Category 3, High Risk
	Patient younger than 40 y Uncomplicated surgery (e.g. hysterectomy) Minimal immobility	General surgery in patient older than 40 y Acute myocardial infarction Chronic illness Leg fracture in a patient younger than 40 y	Hip and major knee surgery Previous venous thrombosis Surgery for extensive malignant disease
Calf vein	approximately 2%	10 - 20%	40 - 70%
Proximal vein thrombosis	approximately 0.4%	2 - 4%	10 - 20%
Fatal pulmonary embolism	< 0.02%	0.2 - 0.5%	1 - 5%

Reprinted with permission from reference 64.

Recommended Prophylaxis for Venous Thromboembolic Disease

Low Risk	Moderate Risk*	High Risk
Early ambulation	Low-dose heparin (5000 U bid) or intermittent pneumatic compression #	LMWH or moderate-dose warfarin or adjusted-dose heparin

* Low-molecular-weight heparin is a reasonable but more expensive option.

Method of choice for neurosurgery, urogenital surgery, or if unusually high risk of hemorrhage (eg, spinal or eye surgery). LMWH indicates low-molecular-weight heparin.

Reprinted with permission from reference 64.

Guidelines for Use of Anticoagulants

Bolus dose of heparin:	5000 U IV
Initial maintenance dose of heparin:	32 000 U IV per 24 h by continuous infusion or 17 000 U subcutaneously to be repeated after adjustment at 12 h

Adjust dose of heparin at 6 h according to nomogram. Maintain aPTT in therapeutic range.

Repeat aPTT 6 times every day until in therapeutic range and then daily (see nomogram).

Start warfarin 10 mg at 24 h and 10 mg next day.

Overlap heparin and warfarin for at least 4 d.

Perform PT daily and adjust warfarin dose to maintain INR at 2.0 to 3.0.

Continue heparin for a minimum of 5 d, then stop if INR has been in therapeutic range for at least 2 consecutive days.

Continue warfarin for 3 mo and monitor PT daily until in therapeutic range, then 3 times during first week, twice weekly for 2 wk, or until dose response is stable, and then every 2 wk.

Obtain a pretreatment hemoglobin level, platelet count, PT, and aPTT and repeat platelet count daily until heparin stopped.

The protocol is modified for patients with large iliofemoral vein thrombi and those with major pulmonary embolus. They are treated with a 7- to 10-day course of heparin and the starting of warfarin therapy is delayed until the aPTT has been in the therapeutic range for 3 days. The delay in starting warfarin is used to ensure that patients receive an adequate dose of heparin for at least 5 days.

aPTT indicates activated partial thromboplastin time; PT, prothrombin time; INR, International Normalized Ratio.

Reprinted with permission from reference 64.

An Intravenous Heparin-Dose Nomogram Based on aPTT Drawn 6 Hours After Starting Heparin*

aPTT (s)	Bolus Dose	Stop Infusion (min)	Rate Change (mL/h) #	Rate Change (U/24 h)	Repeat aPTT
<50	5000 U	0	+3	2880	6 h
50 - 59	0	0	+3	2880	6 h
60 - 85 *	0	0	-2	1920	Next AM
86 - 95	0	0	-2	1920	Next AM
96 - 120	0	30	-4	3840	6 h
> 120	0	60	-4	3840	6 h

* As recommended in Table "Guidelines for Use of Anticoagulants".

\# When infusion fluid 1 mL/h = 40 U/h (ie, 20,000 U heparin in 500 mL).

* PTT equivalent to heparin level of 0.3 - 0.7 U/ml by antifactor Xa assay.

aPTT indicates activated partial thromboplastin time.

Reprinted with permission from reference 64.

Therapeutic Range for Heparin

Test	Therapeutic Range
aPTT	Approximately 1.5 - 3.0 times* mean of laboratory normal range
Heparin level: thrombin/protamine titration	0.2 - 0.4 U/mL
Heparin level: Antifactor Xa	0.3 - 0.7 U/mL

* Depends on sensitivity of aPTT reagents to heparin.
  aPTT indicates activated partial thromboplastin time.

Reprinted with permission from reference 64.

Physiology / Pathophysiology

Renal System

Comparison of Various Crystalloid Solutions

Solution	Dextrose (mg/dl)	Na+ (mEq/L)	Cl- (mEq/L)	K+ (mEq/L)	Mg^{2+} (mEq/L)	Ca^{2+} (mEq/L)	Lactate (mEq/L)	Acetate (mEq/L)	Gluconate (mEq/L)	pH (approx.)	Osmolarity (mOsm/L)
Extracellular Fluid	90-110	140	108	4.5	2.0	5.0	5.0	0	0	7.4	290
Lactated Ringer's	0	130	109	4.0	0	3.0	28	0	0	6.7	273
Plasma-Lyte R	0	140	103	10.0	3.0	5	8	47	0	7.4	312
Plasma-Lyte A	0	140	98	5.0	3.0	0	0	27	23	7.4	294
Isolyte S	0	140	98	5.0	3.0	0	0	27	23	7.4	295
Normosol-R	0	140	98	5.0	3.0	0	0	27	23	7.4	295
0.9% NaCl	0	154	154	0	0	0	0	0	0	5.7	308
5% NaCl	0	855	855	0	0	0	0	0	0	5.6	1171
5% dextrose/water	5000	0	0	0	0	0	0	0	0	5.0	253
5% dextrose/0.45% NaCl	5000	77	77	0	0	0	0	0	0	4.2	405
5% dextrose/0.9% NaCl	5000	154	154	0	0	0	0	0	0	4.2	560
5% dextrose/LR	5000	130	109	4.0	0	3.0	28	0	0	5.3	527
1.5% Glycine	0	0	0	0	0	0	0	0	0	6.0	200
Water, Sterile	0	0	0	0	0	0	0	0	0	5.5	0

Composition of Body Fluids

Source	Na^+ (mEq/liter)	K^+ (mEq/liter)	Cl^- (mEq/liter)	HCO_3 (mEq/liter)	pH	Osmolality (mosm/liter)
Gastric	50	10 - 15	150	0	1	300
Pancreas	140	5	50 - 100	100	9	300
Bile	130	5	100	40	8	300
Ileostomy	130	15 - 20	120	25 - 30	8	300
Diarrhea	50	35	40	50	Alk	
Sweat	50	5	55	0		
Blood	140	4 - 5	100	25	7.4	285 - 295
Urine	0 - 100*	20 - 100*	70 - 100*	0	4.5 - 8.5	50 - 1400

*Varies considerably with intake.

Reprinted with permission from reference 47.

Diagnostic Guide for Serum and Urine Electrolytes

	Serum values					Urine values			
Condition	Na+ (mEq/liter)	K+ (mEq/liter)	Osmolality (mosm/liter)	BUN (mg/dl)	Creatinine	Na+ (mEq/liter)	K+ (mEq/liter)	Osmolality (mosm/liter)	Urea (mg/dl)
Primary aldosteronism	140	↓	280	10	N	80	60 - 80	300 - 800	Low
Secondary aldosteronism	130	↓	275	15 - 25	↓	<20	40 - 60	300 - 400	
Na+ depletion	120-130	N or ↑	260	>30	N or ↑	10 - 20	40	600+	800 - 1000
Na+ overload	150+	N	290+	N or ↑	N	100+	60	500+	300
H_2O overload	120 - 130	↓	260	10 - 15	↓	50 - 80	60	50 - 200	300
Dehydration	150	↓	300	30 or N	N or ↑	40	20 - 40	800+	800 - 1000
Inappropriate ADH	<125	↓	<260	<10	↓	90	60 - 150	$U>P_{Osm}$	300
Acute tubular necrosis									
Oliguric	135	↑	N or ↑	↑↑	↑	40+	20 - 40	300	300
Polyuric	135	N or ↑	275	↑	↑	20	30	300	100 - 300

Reprinted with permission from reference 47.

Differential Diagnosis of Hemoglobinuria and Myoglobinuria

Observation	Hemoglobinuria	Myoglobinuria
Appearance of plasma	Amber to red-brown	Normal[a]
Bilirubin level	Slightly to moderately elevated	Normal
Effect of 80% saturation with ammonium sulfate	Precipitates hemoglobin	Does not precipitate myoglobin (in fresh specimen containing undenatured myoglobin)
Agarose electrophoresis of plasma at pH 8.6	Free plasma hemoglobin migrates near transferrin in β_1 globulin region; addition of haptoglobin[b] moves it into α_2 region; albumin band may appear yellow or brown due to methemalbumin	Myoglobin migrates near C3; addition of haptoglobin[b] has no effect

[a]Except when associated with renal failure.

[b]By addition of normal serum to sample prior to electrophoresis.

Reprinted with permission from reference 61.

Differential Features in Diagnosis of Acute Renal Failure

Parameter	Physiologic oliguria	Prerenal azotemia	Acute tubular necrosis Infant	Adult	Obstructive failure Acute (48 hr)	Chronic (48 hr)
U_{sg}	1024	1016	1010	1000 - 1012	1015 - 1025	1010 - 1015
U_{osm} (mOsm/liter)	750	500	250 - 320	300 - 350	450 - 700	300 - 450
U_{osm}/P_{osm}	2.0	1.5	1.0	1.2	1.5	1.2
Urine flow (ml/kg/hr)	0.25	0.25 - 0.5	Variable	Variable	0.5	1.2
BUN/creat	20:1	20:1	5:1	10:1	20:1	10:1
U_{creat}/P_{creat}	40:1	40:1	10:1	10:1	20 - 40:1	10:1
U_{Na}	10	20	30 - 50	40	20	10 - 50
FE_{Na}	1%	1%	3%	2%	1%	3%
Urine sediment	Protein trace, hyaline casts	Protein trace, hyaline/fine granular casts	Coarse granular casts, hematuria	Renal tubular cells, coarse granular pigmented casts	Protein trace, occasional fine granular casts	Blood trace

Parameter	Physiologic oliguria	Prerenal azotemia	Acute tubular necrosis		Obstructive failure	
			Infant	Adult	Acute (48 hr)	Chronic (48 hr)
Radiology						
Size	Normal	Normal	Variable	Variable	Variable	Small
Nephrogram	Early	Early	Early, dense	Persistent	Delay	Delay
Calyces	Normal.	Normal	Normal	Normal	Dilated	Dilated
Excretion	No delay	Delay	Delay	Delay	Delay	Marked delay
Clinical features	Thirst, mild weight loss loss 2-3%	Circulatory failure, weight	Pain, fever	Dehydration		

Reprinted with permission from reference 64.

Physiology / Pathophysiology

Immune System (including Anaphylaxis)

Differential Diagnosis of Anaphylaxis

Administration of sedative, hypnotic, or anesthetic drugs
Asthma
Cardiogenic shock
Disconnection or overdosage of vasoactive drug infusions
Dysrhythmias
Hereditary angioedema
Jarisch-Herxheimer reactions
Mastocytosis
Pericardial tamponade
Post-extubation stridor
Pulmonary edema
Pulmonary embolus
Septic shock
Tension pneumothorax
Vasovagal reactions
Venous air embolism

Reprinted with permission from reference 66.

Recognition of Anaphylaxis During Regional and General Anesthesia

System	Symptoms	Signs
Respiratory	Dyspnea Chest discomfort	Coughing Wheezing Sneezing Airway obstruction Laryngeal edema Decreased pulmonary compliance Fulminant pulmonary edema Acute respiratory distress
Cardiovascular	Dizziness Malaise Retrosternal oppression	Disorientation Diaphoresis Hypotension Loss of consciousness Tachycardia Dysrhythmias Decreased systemic vascular resistance Pulmonary hypertension Cardiac arrest
Cutaneous	Itching Burning Tingling	Urticaria (hives) Flushing Perioral edema Periorbital edema

Reprinted with permission from reference 66.

Recognition of Anaphylaxis in Intubated Patients

System	Signs
Respiratory	Cyanosis
	Wheezing
	Increased peak airway pressure
	Acute pulmonary edema
Cardiovascular	Tachycardia
	Dysrhythmias
	Hypotension
	Pulmonary hypertension
	Decreased systemic vascular resistance
	Cardiovascular collapse
Cutaneous	Urticaria
	Flushing
	Perioral edema
	Periorbital edema

Reprinted with permission from reference 66.

Drugs Useful in the Therapy for Anaphylaxis

Drug	Receptor Effects	Pharmacologic Effects	Indication
Catecholamines			
Epinephrine	α-agonist	Vasoconstriction	Initial therapy
	β-agonist	Bronchial dilator ↓ Mediator release	
Isoproterenol	β-agonist	Bronchial dilator ↓ Mediator release	Refractory bronchospasm Pulmonary hypertension Right ventricular dysfunction
Norepinephrine	α-agonist β-agonist	↑ Systemic vascular resistance	Refractory hypotension
Phosphodiesterase inhibitors			
Aminophylline		Bronchial dilator ↓ Mediator release	Persistent bronchospasm
Amrinone		Pulmonary vasodilator	Pulmonary hypertension
Enoximone		↑ Inotropy	Right ventricular dysfunction
Milrinone			

Drug	Receptor Effects	Pharmacologic Effects	Indication
Antihistamines			
Diphenhydramine Chlorpheniramine	H_1 antagonist	Competitive inhibition of histamine	All forms of anaphylaxis
Cimetidine Ranitidine Famotidine	H_2 antagonist		Administer with an H_1 antagonist
Corticosteroids			
Hydrocortisone Methylprednisolone		↓ Arachidonic acid metabolites ↑ β-adrenergic effects	Refractory bronchospasm or hypotension Acute late phase reactions

Reprinted with permission from reference 66.

Management of Anaphylaxis

Initial Therapy

1. Stop administration of antigen
2. Maintain airway with 100% oxygen
3. Discontinue all anesthetic agents
4. Start intravascular volume expansion (2 - 4 liters of crystalloid/colloid [25 - 50 ml/kg] with hypotension)
5. Give epinephrine (5 - 10 µg IV with hypotension, titrate as needed; 0.5 to 1 mg IV with cardiovascular collapse)[1]

Secondary Treatment

1. Catecholamine infusions (starting doses):
   Epinephrine 4 - 8 µg/min [0.05-0.1 µg/kg/min][2]
   Norepinephrine 4 - 8 µg/min [0.05-0.1 µg/kg/min][2]
   Isoproterenol 0.5 - 1 µg/min[2]
2. Antihistamines (0.5 - 1 mg/kg diphenhydramine)
3. Corticosteroids (0.25 - 1 g hydrocortisone; alternately 1 - 2 gm [25 mg/kg] methylprednisolone[3]
4. Sodium bicarbonate (0.5 - 1 mEq/kg with persistent hypotension or acidosis)
5. Airway evaluation (prior to extubation)

---

[1]Higher doses may be required if the patient fails to respond or is receiving spinal or epidural anesthesia.

[2]Higher doses may be required.

[3]Methylprednisolone may be the drug of choice if the reaction is suspected to be complement-mediated.

Reprinted with permission from reference 66.

Regional Anesthesia

Sensory Dermatomes in Adults

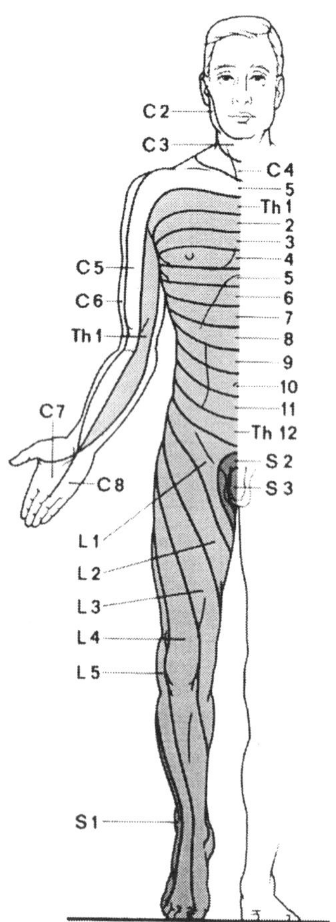

Reprinted with permission from reference 67.

Sensory Dermatomes in Adults

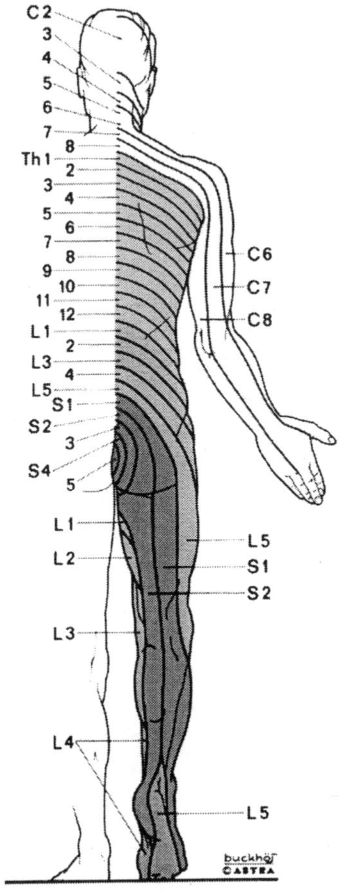

Reprinted with permission from reference 67.

Sensory Dermatomes in Small Infants

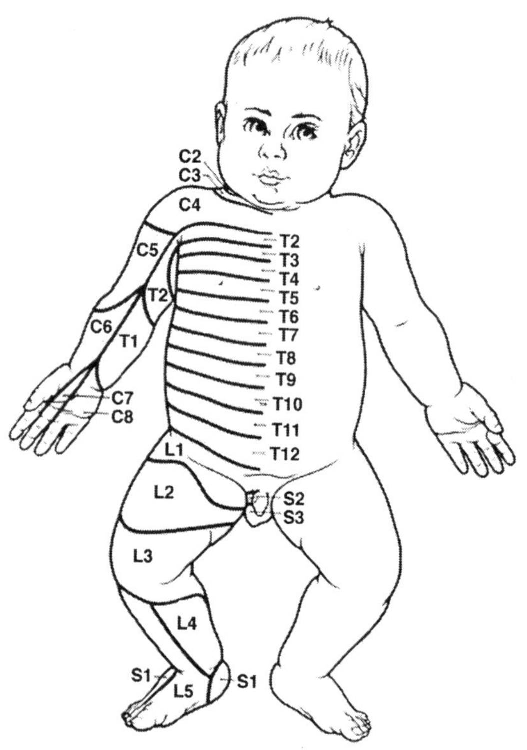

Reprinted with permission from reference 68.

Sensory Dermatomes in Small Infants

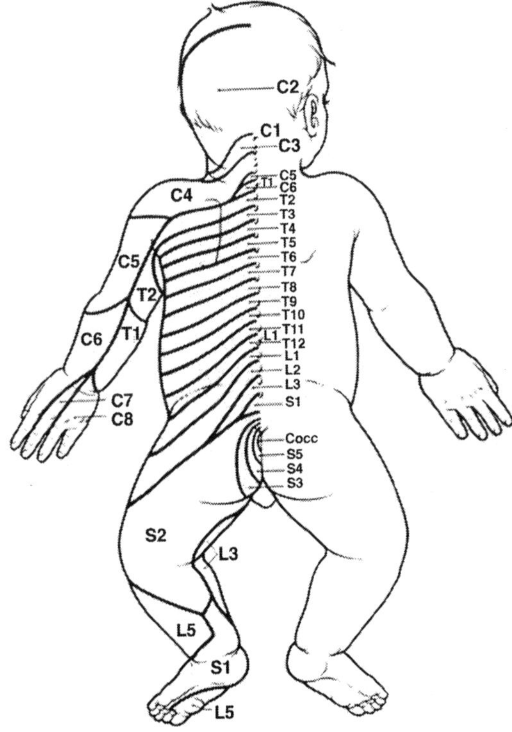

Reprinted with permission from reference 68.

Recommended Levels For Spinal Anesthesia

Operative Site	Level
Lower extremities	T12
Hip	T10
Vagina/uterus	T10
Bladder/prostate	T10
Lower extremities with tourniquet	T8
Testes/ovaries	T8
Lower intra-abdominal	T6
Other intra-abdominal	T4

Tissue Layers Encountered During Epidural/Spinal Blocks

Skin
Supraspinous ligament
Interspinous ligament
Ligamentum flavum
Epidural space (contains loose areolar tissue, fat, and blood vessels)
Dura
"Potential space"
Subarachnoid membrane
Subarachnoid space (lumbar cistern).

Post Dural Puncture Headache

1. Most frequent complication of SAB
2. Etiology - traction on cranial nerves, venous sinuses, or vertebral vessels vs. compensatory venodilation
3. Onset - 90% in 24 - 72 hrs
4. Duration - 80 - 85% < 5 days
5. Postural headache key feature

Complications of Regional Anesthesia

With increasing plasma concentration of local anesthetics, one sees the following:

1. Numbness of tongue
2. Lightheadedness
3. Visual and auditory disturbances
4. Muscular twitches
5. Unconsciousness
6. Convulsions
7. Coma
8. Respiratory arrest
9. Cardiovascular collapse

Peak effect occurs in ~20 min

Intra-arterial dose << intravenous dose of local anesthetic needed to produce toxic effect (e.g., tongue block)

Effect of epinephrine test dose on beta-blocked patient - increased blood pressure with reflex bradycardia

Pregnant female - epinephrine not predictive of intravascular injection - 25 - 50% of patients have increase in heart rate. Is it pain or is it the epinephrine? - Isuprel might be better test drug.

Treatment of Seizures Secondary to Local Anesthetics

1. Thiopental or other induction agent (e.g., propofol)
2. Midazolam or diazepam
3. Succinylcholine

Epinephrine Doses in Local Anesthetics

Dilution	Concentration (μg/ml)
1:1,000	1,000
1:10,000	100
1:100,000	10
1:200,000	5

Try to avoid exceeding 2 μg/kg epinephrine in adults.

Addition of Bicarbonate to Adjust pH of Local Anesthetic Solutions

		HCO_3 (mEq/ 10 mL LA)*	pH after HCO_3
2-Chloroprocaine	2%	1.0	7.47
	3%	1.0	7.43
Mepivacaine	1%	1.0	7.27
	1.5%	0.5	6.98
Bupivacaine	0.25%	0.025	6.97
	0.5%	0.012	6.62
	0.5% with epi	0.075	6.28
Lidocaine	1%	1.0	7.41
	1% with epi	1.0	7.15
	1.5%	1.0	7.26
	1.5% with epi	1.0	7.09
	2%	1.0	7.21
	2% with epi	1.0	7.02

*8% $NaHCO_3$ has 1 mEq/mL of HCO_3; LA = local anesthetic solution

Adapted with permission from reference 69.

Pediatric Anesthesia

Anatomical Differences Between the Neonate and the Adult

Head	Relatively large with prominent occiput
Neck	Short
Tongue	Relatively large which in the absence of teeth fills the oral cavity
Larynx	Narrower, shorter and funnel-shaped, situated more cephalad (C3-4) than in adult (C4-5) with an anterior inclination
Epiglottis	Narrower omega-shaped epiglottis, angled away from the vertical axis of the trachea
Vocal cords	Angled compared with adult
Subglottis	Narrowest at the cricoid ring rather than at the vocal cords as in the adult

Reproduced with permission from reference 70.

Options in Difficult Intubation in Neonates and Small Infants

Simple Methods

- Tongue extraction
- Lateral approach
- Two hands
- Indirect laryngoscopy
- Prone position
- Finger intubation

Complex Methods

- Blind oral intubation ± stylets
- Blind nasal intubation ± stylets
- Retrograde intubation
- Fiberoptic bronchoscope ± guidewire
- Modular semi-disposable flexible endoscopy
- Retrograde-assisted fibreoptic intubation
- Bullard laryngoscope
- Tubular pharyngolaryngoscope
- Light wand intubation
- Laryngeal mask-assisted intubation

Tracheostomy

Adapted with permission from reference 70.

Guidelines for Laryngoscope Blade and Endotracheal Tube Sizes

Age	Suggested Laryngoscope Blade
Neonate and Premature	Miller 0
Up to 6-8 Months	Miller 1
9 Months - 2 Years	Wis-Hipple 1.5, Miller 1
Greater than 2.5 Years	Miller 2, MacIntosh 2

Age	Suggested Endotracheal Tube
Premature-Newborn	2.5-3.0
Full-term Newborn - 9 Months	3.5
12-20 Months	4.0
Over 2 Years	[16 + Age (years)] ÷ 4
French Size	Age (years) + 18

Suggested Endotracheal Tube and Bronchoscope Sizes for Children (by Age)

Age	Cricoid Airway Diameter (mm)	Endotracheal Tube Size (internal diameter, mm)	Distance Inserted from Lips to Place Distal End in the Mid trachea (cm; Add 2-3 cm for Nasal Tube)	Bronchoscope Size
Premature	4.0	2.5 - 3.0	10	2.5
Term newborn	4.5	3.0 - 3.5	11	3.0
6 months	5.0	3.0 - 3.5	11	3.0
1 year	5.5	3.5 - 4.0	12	3.5
2 years	6.0	4.0 - 4.5	13	3.5
3 years	7.0	4.5 - 5.0	14	4.0
5 years	8.0	5.5 - 6.0	15 - 16	5.0
10 years	9.0	6.0 - 6.5	17 - 18	6.0*
12 years	10.0	6.0 - 6.5	18 - 20	6.0*
14 years and older	11.0	7.0 - 8.0	20 - 22	6.0*

*A larger adult-sized bronchoscope may be helpful if there is a large air leak and positive-pressure ventilation is being used

Modified and reproduced with permission from 71.

Clinical Problems in Acute Epiglottitis

Anatomic obstruction
- Edema, inflammation
- Secretions

Respiratory failure
- Hypoxia, respiratory acidosis

Fatigue (depends on length and severity of increased respiratory effort)

Circulatory status
- Dehydration → metabolic acidosis

Toxic and febrile
- Increased oxygen demand

Decreased central nervous system function

Reproduced with permission from reference 72.

Differential Diagnosis of Laryngotracheobronchitis and Epiglottitis

	Epiglottitis	Croup
Etiology	Bacterial	Viral*
Age	1 year - adult	1 - 5 years
Obstruction	Supraglottic	Subglottic
Onset	Sudden (hours)	Gradual (days)
Fever	High	Low grade
Dysphagia	Marked	None
Drooling	Present	Minimal
Posture	Sitting	Recumbent
Toxemia	Mild → severe	Mild
Cough	Usually none	Barking, brassy
Voice	Clear to muffled	Hoarse
Respiratory rate	Normal → rapid	Rapid
Larynx palpation	Tender	Not tender
White Blood Cell count	High (>18,000)	Usually normal
Clinical course	Shorter	Longer
Most common source	H. influenza (children) Group A Strep (adults)	Parainfluenza virus

*Occasionally complicated by bacterial tracheitis (pseudomembranous croup)

Reproduced with permission from reference 72.

Neonatal Resuscitation Supplies and Equipment

Suction Equipment

Bulb syringe
Mechanical suction
Suction catheters, 5F or 6F, 8F, 10F
8F feeding tube and 20-mL syringe
Meconium aspirator

Bag-and-Mask Equipment

Neonatal resuscitation bag with a pressure-release valve or pressure gauge - the bag must be capable of delivering 90% to 100% oxygen. Face masks, newborn and premature sizes (cushioned rim masks preferred)
Oral airways, newborn and premature sizes
Oxygen with flowmeter and tubing

Intubation Equipment

Laryngoscope with straight blades, No. 0 (preterm) and No. 1 (term)
Extra bulbs and batteries for laryngoscope
Endotracheal tubes, 2.5, 3.0, 3.5, 4.0 mm
Stylet
Scissors
Gloves

Medications

Epinephrine 1:10,000 - 3-mL or 10-mL ampules
Naloxone hydrochloride 0.4 mg/mL - 1-mL ampules, or
1.0 mg/mL - 2-mL ampules
Volume expander, one or more of these:
—5% Albumin-saline solution
—Normal saline
—Ringer's lactate
Sodium bicarbonate 4.2% (5 mEq/10 mL) - 10-mL ampules
Dextrose 10%, 250 mL
Sterile water, 30 mL
Normal saline, 30 mL

Miscellaneous

Radiant warmer
Stethoscope
Cardiotachometer with ECG (oscilloscope desirable)
Adhesive tape, 1/2 or 3/4 inch
Syringes, 1, 3, 5, 10, 20, 50 mL
Needles, 25, 21, 18 gauge
Alcohol sponges
Umbilical artery catheterization tray
Umbilical tape
Umbilical catheters, 3.5F, 5F
Three-way stopcocks
Feeding tube, 5F

Pediatric Resuscitation Drugs

Drug	How Supplied	Dose (µg or mEq)	Dose (ml)	Frequency
Atropine	0.4 mg/ml	0.01 - 0.03 mg/kg	0.025 - 0.075 ml/kg	20 min
Calcium chloride	100 mg/ml (10%) (27 mg Ca^{2+}/ml)	30 mg/kg (8 mg Ca^{2+}/kg)	0.3 ml/kg	10 - 20 min
Calcium gluconate	100 mg/ml (10%) (9 mg Ca^{2+}/ml)	100 mg/kg (9 mg Ca^{2+}/kg)	1.0 ml/kg	10 - 20 min
Dopamine	40 mg/ml	2 - 10 µg/kg/min	--	Infusion
Epinephrine	0.1 mg/ml (1:10,000)	1 - 5 µg/kg for hypotension 10 - 100 µg/kg for cardiac arrest	0.01 - 0.05 ml/kg 0.1 - 0.1 ml/kg	5 min
	1 mg/ml (1:1,000)	1 - 5 µg/kg for hypotension 10 - 100 µg/kg for cardiac arrest	0.001 - 0.005 ml/kg 0.01 - 0.01 ml/kg	
Isoproterenol	0.2 mg/ml	0.1 - 1.5 µg/kg/min	--	Infusion
Lidocaine	10 mg/ml (1%)	1 mg/kg 20 - 50 µg/kg/min	0.1 ml/kg --	5 - 10 min Infusion
Sodium bicarbonate	1 mEq/ml	1 - 2 mEq/kg, or 0.3 x kg x base deficit	1 - 2 ml/kg	10 min, or by ABGs
Naloxone	0.02 mg/ml 0.4 mg/ml	0.01 mg/kg	0.5 ml/kg 0.025 ml/kg	2 - 5 min
Defibrillation	--	2 watt-sec/kg; may double and repeat		prn

Medications for Neonatal Resuscitation

Medication	Concentration to Administer	Preparation	Dosage/ Route*	Total Dose/Infant: Weight	Total Dose	Total mL	Rate/Precautions
Epinephrine	1:10,000	1 mL	0.1 - 0.3 mL/kg	1 kg		0.1 - 0.3 mL	Give rapidly
				2 kg		0.2 - 0.6 mL	May dilute with normal saline to 1 - 2 mL if giving by ET
				3 kg		0.3- 0.9 mL	
			IV or ET	4 kg		0.4 - 1.2 mL	
Volume Expanders	Whole blood 5% Albumin-saline Normal saline Ringer's lactate	40 mL IV	10 mL/kg	1 kg		10 mL	Give over 5 - 10 minutes
				2 kg		20 mL	
				3 kg		30 mL	
				4 kg		40 mL	
Sodium Bicarbonate	0.5 mEq/mL (4.2% solution)	20 mL or two 10-mL prefilled syringes	2 mEq/kg IV	1 kg	2 mEq	4 mL	Give *slowly*, over at least 2 minutes
				2 kg	4 mEq	8 mL	Give only if infant is being effectively ventilated
				3 kg	6 mEq	12 mL	
				4 kg	8 mEq	16 mL	

Medication	Concentration to Administer	Preparation	Dosage/ Route*	Total Dose/Infant			Rate/Precautions
				Weight	**Total Dose**	**Total mL**	
Naloxone Hydrochloride	0.4 mg/mL	1 mL	0.1 mg/kg	1 kg	0.1 mg	0.25 mL	Give rapidly
			(0.25 mL/kg)	2 kg	0.2 mg	0.50 mL	IV, ET preferred
			IV, ET	3 kg	0.3 mg	0.75 mL	IM, SQ acceptable
			IM, SQ	4 kg	0.4 mg	1.00 mL	
	1.0 mg/mL	1 mL	0.1 mg/kg	1 kg	0.1 mg	0.1 mL	Give rapidly
			(0.1 mL/kg)	2 kg	0.2 mg	0.2 mL	IV, ET preferred
			IV, ET	3 kg	0.3 mg	0.3 mL	IM, SQ acceptable
			IM, SQ	4 kg	0.4 mg	0.4 mL	
				Weight	**Total µg/min**		
Dopamine	$\frac{6 \times \text{Weight (kg)} \times \text{Desired dose } (\mu g/kg/min)}{\text{Desired fluid (mL/h)}}$ =	mg of dopamine per 100 mL of solution	Begin at 5 µg/kg/min (may increase to 20 µg/kg/min if necessary)	1 kg	5 - 20 µg/min		Give as a continuous infusion using an infusion pump
				2 kg	10 - 40 µg/min		Monitor heart rate and blood pressure closely
				3 kg	15- 60 µg/min		Seek consultation
				4 kg	20 - 80 µg/min		

*IM, intramuscular; ET, endotracheal; IV, intravenous; SQ, subcutaneous

Reprinted with permission from reference 73.

Normal Blood Gas Values in the Newborn

Subject	Age	pO2 (mmHg)	pCO2 (mmHg)	pH	Base Excess (mEq/L)
Fetus (term)	Before labor	25	40	7.37	-2
Fetus (term)	End of labor	10-20	55	7.25	-5
Newborn (term)	10 minutes	50	48	7.20	-10
Newborn (term)	1 hour	70	35	7.35	-5
Newborn (term)	1 week	75	35	7.40	-2
Newborn (preterm, 1,500 gm)	1 week	60	38	7.37	-3

Reproduced with permission from reference 74.

Normal and Acceptable Hematocrits in Pediatric Patients

	Normal Hematocrit Mean	Range	Acceptable Hematocrit
Premature	45	40 - 50	35 - 40
Newborn	54	45 - 65	35 - 40
3 months	36	*30 - 42**	25
1 year	38	34 - 42	20 - 25
6 years	38	35 - 43	20 - 25

Reproduced with permission from reference 74.

*Note that 3 months is the physiologic nadir for the hematocrit.

Evaluation of Severity of Dehydration

Examination	Older Child: 3% Infant: 5%	6% 10%	9% 15%
Skin turgor	Normal	Tenting	None
Skin-touch	Normal	Dry	Clammy
Buccal mucosa/lips	Moist	Dry	Parched/cracked
Eyes	Normal	Deep-set	Sunken
Crying-tears	Present	Reduced	None
Fontanelle	Flat	Soft	Sunken
CNS	Consolable	Irritable	Lethargic
Pulse	Regular	Slight increased	Tachycardia
Urine output	Normal	Decreased	Anuria

Reprinted with permission from reference 75.

Guidelines for Fluid Administration in Pediatric Patients: Balanced Salt Solution

1. First hour: hydrating solution
   - Age 3 and under: 25 ml/kg, plus item 4 below
   - Age 4 and over: 20 ml/kg, plus item 4 below

2. Maintenance fluid requirements for all other hours, plus item 4 below

First 10 kg	= 4 ml/kg/hr
Second 10 kg	= 2 ml/kg/hr
Greater than 20 kg	= 1 ml/kg/hr

3. Hourly fluid beyond maintenance fluid requirements

Mild trauma	= 2 ml/kg/hr
Moderate trauma	= 4 ml/kg/hr
Maximal trauma	= 6 ml/kg/hr

4. Blood replacement with blood or 3:1 volume replacement with balanced salt solution

Adapted with permission from reference 74.

Definitions of Hypertension in Children

Term	Definition
Normal BP	Systolic and diastolic BPs <90th percentile for age and sex
High normal BP*	Average systolic and/or average diastolic BP between 90th and 95th percentiles for age and sex
High BP (hypertension)	Average systolic and/or average diastolic BPs ≥95th percentile for age and sex with measurements obtained on at least three occasions

* If the BP reading is high normal for age, but can be accounted for by excess height for age or excess lean body mass for age, such children are considered to have normal BP.

Reprinted with permission from reference 14.

Classification of Hypertension in Children by Age Group

Age Group	Significant Hypertension (mm Hg)	Severe Hypertension (mm Hg)
Newborn		
7 day	Systolic BP ≥96	Systolic BP ≥106
8 - 30 day	Systolic BP ≥104	Systolic BP ≥110
Infant (<2 yr)	Systolic BP ≥112 Diastolic BP ≥74	Systolic BP ≥118 Diastolic BP ≥82
Children (3-5 yr)	Systolic BP ≥116 Diastolic BP ≥76	Systolic BP ≥124 Diastolic BP ≥84
Children (6-9 yr)	Systolic BP ≥122 Diastolic BP ≥78	Systolic BP ≥130 Diastolic BP ≥86
Children (10-12 yr)	Systolic BP ≥126 Diastolic BP ≥82	Systolic BP ≥134 Diastolic BP ≥90
Adolescents (13-15 yr)	Systolic BP ≥136 Diastolic BP ≥86	Systolic BP ≥144 Diastolic BP ≥92
Adolescents (16-18 yr)	Systolic BP ≥142 Diastolic BP ≥92	Systolic BP ≥150 Diastolic BP ≥98

Modified with permission from reference 14.

Age-Specific Percentiles of Blood Pressure Measurements in Boys - Birth to 12 Months

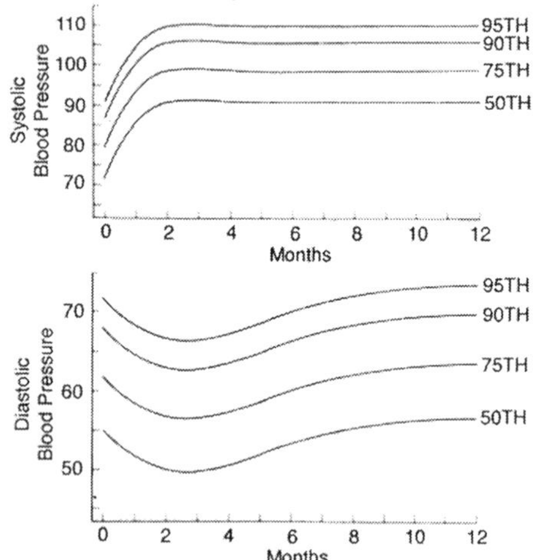

(90th Percentile)

Age (Months)	Systolic BP	Diastolic BP	Height (cm)	Weight (kg)
0	87	68	51	4
1	101	65	59	4
2	106	63	63	5
3	106	63	66	5
4	106	63	68	6
5	105	65	70	7
6	105	66	72	8
7	105	67	73	9
8	105	68	74	9
9	105	68	76	10
10	105	69	77	10
11	105	69	78	11
12	105	69	80	11

Korotkoff phase IV (K4) used for diastolic BP

Modified with permission from reference 14.

Age-Specific Percentiles of Blood Pressure Measurements in Girls - Birth to 12 Months

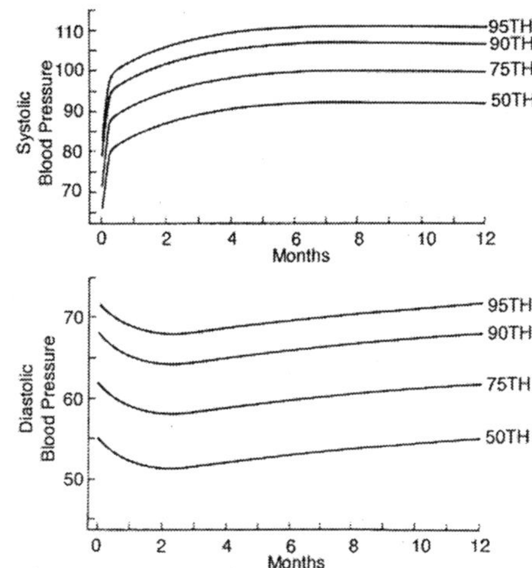

(90th Percentile)

Age (Months)	Systolic BP	Diastolic BP	Height (cm)	Weight (kg)
0	78	68	54	4
1	98	65	55	4
2	101	64	56	4
3	104	64	58	5
4	105	65	61	5
5	106	65	63	6
6	106	66	66	7
7	106	66	68	8
8	106	66	70	9
9	106	67	72	9
10	106	67	74	10
11	105	67	75	10
12	105	67	77	11

Korotkoff phase IV (K4) used for diastolic BP

Modified with permission from reference 14.

Age-Specific Percentiles of Blood Pressure Measurements in Boys - 1 to 13 Years

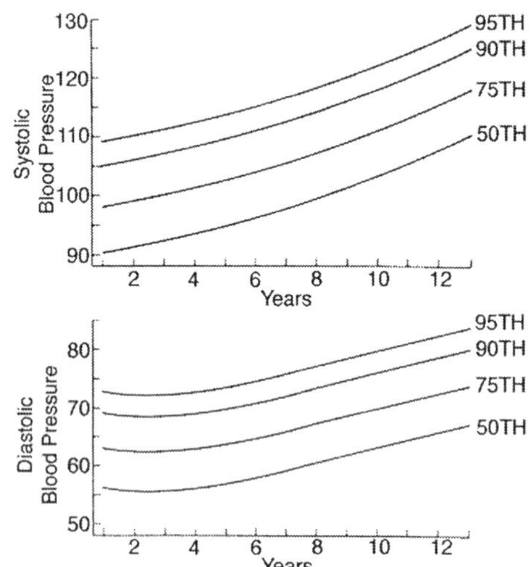

(90th Percentile)

Age (Years)	Systolic BP	Diastolic BP	Height (cm)	Weight (kg)
1	105	69	80	11
2	106	68	91	14
3	107	68	100	16
4	108	69	108	18
5	109	69	115	22
6	111	70	122	25
7	112	71	129	29
8	114	73	135	34
9	115	74	141	39
10	117	75	147	44
11	119	76	153	50
12	121	77	159	55
13	124	79	165	62

Korotkoff phase IV (K4) used for diastolic BP

Modified with permission from reference 14.

Age-Specific Percentiles of Blood Pressure Measurements in Girls - 1 to 13 Years

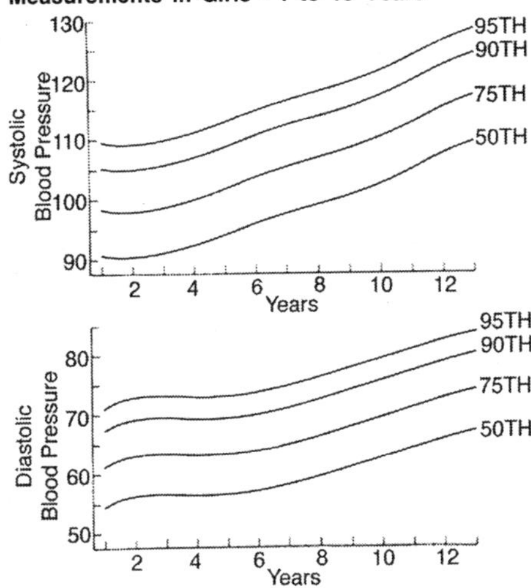

(90th Percentile)

Age (Years)	Systolic BP	Diastolic BP	Height (cm)	Weight (kg)
1	105	67	77	11
2	105	69	89	13
3	106	69	98	15
4	107	69	107	18
5	109	69	115	22
6	111	70	122	25
7	112	71	129	30
8	114	72	135	35
9	115	74	142	40
10	117	75	148	45
11	119	77	154	51
12	122	78	160	58
13	124	80	165	63

Korotkoff phase IV (K4) used for diastolic BP

Modified with permission from reference 14.

Age-Specific Percentiles of Blood Pressure Measurements in Boys - 13 to 18 Years

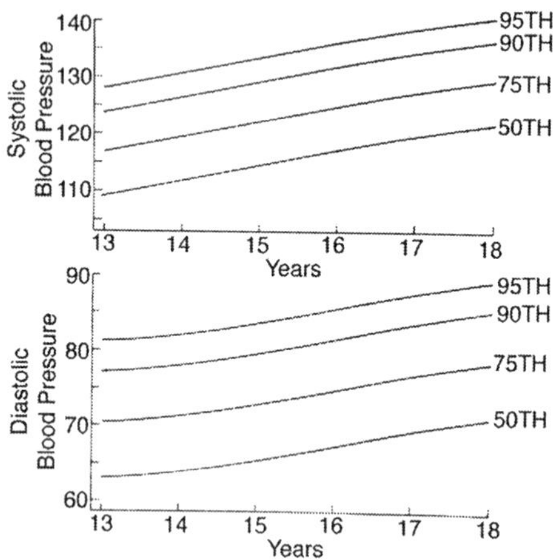

(90th Percentile)

Age (Years)	Systolic BP	Diastolic BP	Height (cm)	Weight (kg)
13	124	77	165	62
14	126	78	172	68
15	129	79	178	74
16	131	81	182	80
17	134	83	184	84
18	136	84	184	86

Korotkoff phase IV (K4) used for diastolic BP

Modified with permission from reference 14.

Age-Specific Percentiles of Blood Pressure Measurements in Girls - 13 to 18 Years

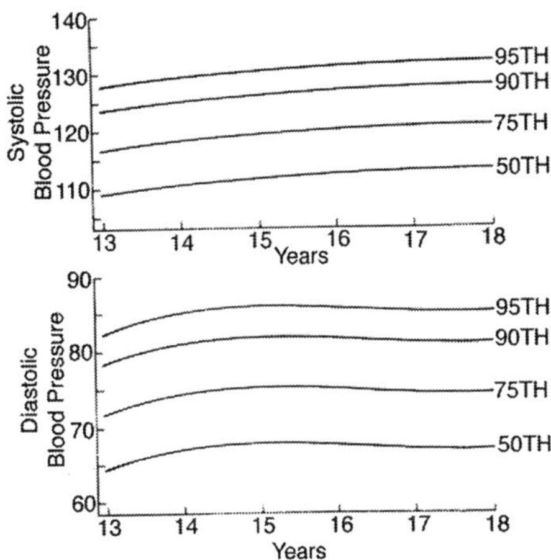

(90th Percentile)

Age (Years)	Systolic BP	Diastolic BP	Height (cm)	Weight (kg)
13	124	78	165	63
14	125	81	166	67
15	126	82	169	70
16	127	81	170	72
17	127	80	170	73
18	127	80	170	74

Korotkoff phase IV (K4) used for diastolic BP

Modified with permission from reference 14.

An Index of Syndromes and Their Anesthetic Implications

Patients often present for anesthesia and surgery having been "labeled" with a diagnosis of some eponymous or rare syndrome. This index is an attempt to catalogue as many syndromes as possible which have anesthetic implications and to give an indication of their main features. It is hoped that it will be useful as a ready reference especially for those involved in pediatric anesthesia, as many of these patients present in infancy or childhood. The information is presented in tabular form with a cross index of alternative names.

Name	*Description*	*Anesthetic Implications*
Adrenogenital syndrome	Inability to synthesize hydrocortisone. Virilization of female	All need hydrocortisone even if not salt-losing. Check electrolytes
Albers-Schonberg disease (marble bone disease or osteopetrosis)	Brittle bones, pathological fractures	Anemia from marrow sclerosis. Hepatosplenomegaly. Care in positioning and restraint.
Albright-Butler syndrome	Renal tubular acidosis, hypokalemia. Renal calculi	Correct electrolytes to within normal limits. Renal impairment
Albright's osteodystrophy (pseudohypoparathyroidism)	Ectopic bone formation. Mental retardation	Hypocalcemia - possible ECG conduction defects, neuromuscular problems. Convulsions
Alport syndrome	Nephritis and nerve deafness. Renal pathology variable	Renal failure in 2nd - 3rd decade. Care with renally excreted drugs
Alstrom syndrome	Obesity, blindness by seven years. Hearing loss. Diabetes after puberty - glomerulosclerosis.	Renal impairment. Management of diabetes and obesity

Analbuminemia	Almost absent albumin 4-100 mg/dl	Very sensitive to protein bound drugs including thiopental, coumarin anticoagulants, curare
Aperts syndrome (acrocephalosyndactyly)	Craniosynostosis	Difficult intubation. Possibly raised intracranial pressure, associated congenital heart disease
Arthrogryposis multiplex	Multiple congenital contractures	Ten percent have congenital heart disease. Minimal thiopental required - muscles replaced by fat. Possible airway problem with mandible.
Asplenia syndrome	Absent spleen, bilateral visceral right sidedness	Very complex cardiovascular anomalies, present with cyanosis and heart failure
Ataxia-telangiectasia	Cerebellar ataxia. Skin and conjunctival telangiectasia. Decreased serum IgA and IgE. 10 percent develop reticuloendothelial malignancy	Defective immunity - recurrent chest and sinus infections. Bronchiectasis
Beckwith syndrome (infantile gigantism)	Birth weight > 4,000 gm. Macroglossia and omphalocele	Persistent severe neonatal hypoglycemia. Airway problems
Bowen's syndrome (cerebrohepatorenal syndrome)	Hepatomegaly and neonatal jaundice. Polycystic kidneys. Associated congenital heart disease. Muscular hypotonia	Hypoprothrombinemia. Care with renally excreted drugs and muscle relaxants

Name	Description	Anesthetic Implications
Carpenter's syndrome	Cranial synostosis. Associated congenital heart disease	Hypoplastic mandible. Possibly difficult intubation
Central core disease	Muscular dystrophy	See myotonia congenita
Chediak-Higashi syndrome	Partial albinism, immunodeficiency, hepatosplenomegaly	Steroid therapy. Recurrent chest infection. Thrombocytopenia - may require platelets
Cherubism	Tumorous lesion of mandibles and maxillae with intraoral masses. May cause respiratory distress	Intubation may be extremely difficult. May require tracheostomy for acute respiratory distress. Profuse bleeding at surgery
Chotzen syndrome	Craniosynostosis	May be difficult intubation. Associated renal anomalies and possible impaired renal excretion of drugs
Christ-Siemens Touraine syndrome (anhidrotic ectodermal dysplasia)	Absent sweating - heat intolerance	Cannot control temperature by sweating. Persistent upper respiratory and chest infection due to poor mucus formation
Chronic granulomatous disease	Inherited disorder of leukocyte function. Recurrent infections with non-pathogenic organisms	Hepatomegaly in 95 percent. Poor pulmonary function. Avoid infection - strict asepsis.

Conradi's syndrome	Chondrodystrophy with contractures, saddle nose, mental retardation. Associated congenital heart disease and renal anomalies	Problems are those of associated renal and cardiac disease
Cretinism (congenital hypothyroidism)	Absent thyroid tissue or defective synthesis thyroxine and goiter	Airway problems - large tongue, goiter. Respiratory center very sensitive to depression. CO_2 retention common. Hypoglycemia, hyponatremia, hypotension. Low cardiac output. Transfusion poorly tolerated.
Cri-Du-Chat syndrome	Chromosome 5-P abnormal. Abnormal cry, microcephaly micrognathia. Congenital heart disease	Airway problems - stridor, laryngomalacia. Possibly difficult intubation
Crouzon disease	Craniosynostosis	Possibly difficult intubation. Severe blood loss with cranial operation
Cutis laxa	Elastic fiber degeneration, pendulous skin, frequent hernias. Emphysema and cor pulmonale. Arterial fragility	Pulmonary infection, emphysema and cor pulmonale. Poor tissues - IV difficult to maintain. Excess of soft tissues around larynx may lead to respiratory obstruction
Down's syndrome (mongolism)	Microcephaly. Small nasopharynx. Hypotonia. Sixty percent have congenital heart disease. Duodenal atresia in some. Cervical spine abnormalities	Difficult airway - large tongue, small mouth. Risk of laryngeal spasm especially on extubation. Problems of cardiac anomalies

Name	Description	Anesthetic Implications
Duchenne muscular dystrophy	Muscular dystrophy with frequent cardiac muscle involvement. Usually die in 2nd decade. Amount of skeletal muscle involvement and cardiac involvement unrelated.	As for myotonia congenita plus cardiac involvement. Minimal drug dosage. Avoid respiratory depressants, muscle relaxants. Post-operative ventilatory support may be required.
Edward's syndrome (Trisomy 18(E))	Congenital heart disease in 95 percent. Micrognathia in 80 percent. Renal malformations 50-80 percent. Usually die in infancy	Possible difficult intubation. Care with renally excreted drugs
Ehlers-Danlos syndrome	Collagen abnormality with hyperelasticity and fragile tissues. Dissecting aneurysm of aorta. Fragility of other blood vessels. Bleeding diathesis - ? cause	CVS - spontaneous rupture of vessels. Angiogram 1 percent mortality. ECG conduction abnormalities. IV difficult to maintain - hematoma. Poor tissues and clotting defects lead to hemorrhage especially GI tract. Spontaneous pneumothorax
Ellis-Van-Creveld syndrome (Chondroectodermal dysplasia)	Ectodermal defects, skeletal anomalies. 50 percent have congenital heart disease, usually septal	Chest wall anomalies lead to poor lung function. May have abnormal maxilla and upper lip, hepatosplenomegaly
Fabry's disease	Lipid storage disease	CVS - hypertension, myocardial ischemia (before 3rd or 4th decade). Renal failure - care with renally excreted drugs

Familial periodic paralysis	Muscle disease. Hypokalemia, attacks of quadriplegia	Monitor serum K^+. Limit use of dextrose Monitor ECG. Avoid relaxants
Fanconi syndrome (renal tubular acidosis)	Usually 2° to other disease. Proximal tubular defect. Acidosis, K^+ loss, dehydration	Impaired renal function. Treat electrolyte and acid-base abnormalities. Look for 1° disease (galactosemia, cysteinosis, etc.)
Farber's disease (lipogranulomatosis)	Sphingomyelin deposition. Widespread visceral lipogranulomas especially in the central nervous system	Deposits in larynx - careful intubation. Generalized systemic involvement leading to cardiac, renal failure
Favism	G-6-P-D deficiency, Hemolytic anemia	Hemolysis following oxidant drugs, (e.g. ASA and sulfa drugs). Anemia - transfuse if necessary
Freidreich's ataxia	Degeneration of cerebellum, lateral and posterior column of spinal cord. Scoliosis. Myocardial degeneration and fibrosis	Heart failure and arrhythmias. Care with cardiac depressant drugs
Gardner's syndrome	Multiple polyposis, bony tumors, sebaceous cysts, fibromas	No anesthetic problems described
Glanzmann's disease (thrombasthenia)	Platelet ADP, reduced - abnormal function	No specific therapy for bleeding. Platelet transfusion disappointing. History of steroids
Goldenhar syndrome (oculo-auriculo-vertebral syndrome)	Unilateral facial hypoplasia. Congenital heart disease in 20 percent. Sixty percent mandibular hypoplasia	Difficult airway and intubation. Problems of associated cardiac disease

Name	***Description***	***Anesthetic Implications***
Goltz-Gorlin syndrome (focal dermal hypoplasia)	Herniae, prolapse, etc. Congenital heart disease - AS or ASD. Renal anomalies	Asymmetry of head - difficult airway
Gorlin syndrome	Basal cell nevi, skeletal anomalies	No anesthetic problem described
Groenblad-Strandberg (pseudoxanthoma elasticum)	Degeneration elastic tissue in skin, eye and cardiovascular system	Rupture of arteries, especially GI tract, hypertension, arterial calcification. Occlusion of cerebral and coronary, arteries. Difficult maintenance of IV cannula
Guillain-Barre syndrome (acute idiopathic polyneuritis)	Acute polyneuropathy. Progressive peripheral neuritis often involving cranial nerves, bulbar palsy with hypoventilation and hypotension	Avoid succinylcholine for at least 3 months - K^+ release. May require tracheostomy and IPPV, support of blood pressure
Hermansky syndrome	Albinism, bleeding diathesis	Platelet abnormality. Try platelet transfusion. No specific treatment
Homocystinuria	Inborn error of metabolism. Thromboembolic phenomena due to intimal thickening. Ectopia lentis, osteoporosis, kyphoscoliosis	Dextran-70 to reduce viscosity and platelet adhesiveness, increase peripheral perfusion. Angiography may precipitate thrombosis especially cerebral

Hunter syndrome (mucopolysaccharidosis II)	Stiff joints, dwarfing, hepatosplenomegaly. Pectus excavatum and kyphoscoliosis. Valvular and coronary heart disease	Upper airway obstruction due to infiltration of lymphoid tissue and larynx. Pneumonias. Possible hypersplenism. Cardiac failure.
Hurler syndrome (mucopolysaccharidosis I)	Pulmonary hypertension. Usually die before ten years from respiratory and cardiac failure	As for Hunter, but more severe. Frequent upper respiratory infection. Abnormal tracheobronchial cartilages. Severe coronary artery disease at early age, valvular and myocardial involvement.
Jervell-Nielson syndrome (cardio-auditory syndrome)	Cardiac conduction defects. Deafness	Syncope, arrhythmias. ECG-large T waves prolonged QT. May need digoxin and/or propranolol or pacemaker
Kartagener's syndrome	Dextrocardia, sinusitis and bronchiectasis. Abnormal immunity. See Asplenia syndrome	Chronic respiratory infection
Klinefelter syndrome (gonosomal aneuploidy)	Tall stature, reduced intelligence. Vertebral collapse due to osteoporosis	No described anesthetic problem. Care in positioning
Klippel-Feil syndrome	Congenital fusion two or more cervical vertebrae leading to neck rigidity	Difficult airway and intubation
Klippel-Trenaunay syndrome (angio-osteohypertrophy)	Usually unilateral. Arteriovenous fistulae thrombocytopenia	Arteriovenous fistulae and anemia lead to high cardiac output state. Thrombocytopenia in visceral hemangiomata

Name	Description	Anesthetic Implications
Laurence-Moon-Biedl syndrome	Obesity, retinitis pigmentosa. Polydactyly. Mental retardation	May be associated with cardiac defects, renal disease and occasionally diabetes insipidus
Larsens syndrome	Multiple congenital dislocations. Connective tissue defect. Poor cartilage in rib cage, epiglottis, arytenoids	Possible difficult intubation. Chronic respiratory problems
Leopard syndrome	Multiple large freckles. Congenital heart disease. ECG anomalies - aberrant conduction. Hypertelarism	Ninety-five percent pulmonary stenosis
Leprechaunism	Failure to thrive, endocrine disorders, severe mental retardation	Hypoglycemia due to hyperinsulinism from hyperplastic Islets of Langerhans. Renal tubular defects - impaired renal function
Letterer-Siwe disease (histiocytosis X)	Histiocytic granulomata in viscera and bones. Clinical course similar to acute leukemia	Pancytopenia-anemia and purpura hemorrhage. Pulmonary infiltration. Hepatic involvement. Gingival inflammation and necrosis, loss of teeth
Median cleft face syndrome	Varying degrees of cleft face. Frontal lipomas, dermoids	Cleft nose, lip and palate may cause intubation difficulties

Lipodystrophy (total lipoatrophy)	Generalized loss all body fat. Fatty, fibrotic liver. Portal hypertension and splenomegaly. Nephropathy. Diabetes	Liver failure - avoid halothane and drugs metabolized by liver. Hypersplenism - anemia and thrombocytopenia. Possible renal failure. Usual diabetic precautions
Lowe syndrome (oculocerebrorenal syndrome)	Male only. Cataract, glaucoma. Mental retardation. Hypotonia. Renal acidosis, proteinuria, osteoporosis and rickets	Check electrolyte and acid-base balance. Check serum Ca^{++} (treated with Vit. D and Ca^{++}). Care with renally excreted drugs
Maffucci syndrome	Enchondromatosis and hemangiomata with malignant change	Pathological fractures. GI bleeding from hemangiomata. Orthostatic hypotension. May be sensitive to vasodilator drugs
Maple-Syrup urine disease (branched chain ketonuria)	Amino acid disturbance treated by diet only. Severe neurological damage and respiratory disturbances	General supportive measures
Marfan's syndrome (arachnodactyly)	Connective tissue disorder. Dilated aortic root leads to AI. Aortic, thoracic or abdominal aneurysm. Pulmonary artery, mitral valve involved. Kyphoscoliosis, pectus excavatum, lung cysts. Joint instability and dislocation	Care with myocardial depressant drugs. Beware possible dissection of aorta. Lung function poor. Possible pneumothorax. Care in positioning - easily dislocated joints
Meckel's syndrome	Microcephaly, micrognathia and cleft epiglottis. Congenital heart disease. Renal dysplasia	Intubation may be difficult. Cardiac problems. Renal failure in infancy - care with renally excreted drugs

Name	Description	Anesthetic Implications
Median cleft face syndrome	Varying degrees of cleft face. Frontal lipomas, dermoids	Cleft nose, lip and palate may cause intubation difficulties
Mobius syndrome (congenital facial diplegia)	Associated limb deformities, micrognathia	Feeding difficulties and aspiration may cause chronic pulmonary problems. May be difficult to intubate
Morquio-Ullrich syndrome (mucopolysaccharidosis IV)	Severe dwarfing. Aortic incompetence. Thoracic deformities. Unstable atlanto-axial joint	Cardiorespiratory symptoms by 2nd decade. Severe kyphoscoliosis with poor lung function. All develop spinal cord damage from atlanto-occipital subluxation
Moschkowitz disease (thrombotic thrombocytopenic purpura)	Hemolytic anemia and thrombocytopenia. Small vessel disease. Neurologic damage and renal disease. Treatment - splenectomy and steroids	History of steroid therapy. Care with renally excreted drugs if kidneys affected
Myasthenia congenita	Like adult myasthenia gravis	Avoid respiratory depressants, muscle relaxants. May require post-op IPPV. Problems with anticholinesterase therapy pre- and post-op. Possibility of cholinergic crisis
Myotonia congenita (Thomsens disease)	Decreased ability to relax muscles after contraction. Diffuse hypertrophy of muscle	Avoid relaxants and depressants, as for Myotonic Dystrophy, though this is a more benign disease, non progressive

Myotonic dystrophy (myotonia dystrophica)	Weakness, myotonia, ptosis, cataracts, partial baldness and gonadal atrophy. Cardiac conduction defects and arrhythmias. Impaired ventilation	Avoid succinylcholine which causes myotonia in 50 percent. Nondepolarizing drugs do not relax myotonia. Neostigmine induces myotonia. Monitor ECG. Extremely sensitive to respiratory depressants, use regional or inhalational agents. IPPV post-op if necessary. Halothane may cause post-op shivering and myotonia. Pulmonary complications due to poor cough
McArdle disease	Glycogen storage disease V	Muscles affected including cardiac muscle: care with cardiac depressant drugs
Neonatal hypoglycemia (idiopathic)	Symptomatic hypoglycemia in infancy - convulsions, lethargy and mental retardation if untreated. No ketosis. Therapy subtotal pancreatectomy	Extreme care in monitoring blood glucose. Steroids, diazoxide and glucagon as required. After pancreatectomy may require insulin and glucose to maintain blood sugar in normal limits
Noack's syndrome	Craniosynostosis and digital anomalies. Obesity	May be difficult to intubate because of skull deformity
Noonan syndrome (male Turner syndrome)	Short stature, mental retardation, congenital heart disease, micrognathia. Hydronephrosis or hypoplasia of kidneys	Usually pulmonary stenosis or PDA, tetralogy, ASD. Care with renally excreted drugs if kidneys affected

Name	Description	Anesthetic Implications
Olliers syndrome (enchondromatosis)	Multiple chondromata within bones, usually unilateral. Pathological fractures	With cavernous hemangioma is described as Maffucci syndrome. Care with positioning
Oro-facial-digital syndrome	Cleft lip and palate, lobed tongue. Hypoplastic mandible and maxilla. Digital anomalies. Hydrocephalus, polycystic kidneys	Difficult airway and intubation. Possible renal failure - care with renally excreted drugs
Osler-Weber-Rendu syndrome (hemorrhagic telangiectasia)	No coagulation abnormalities. Associated pulmonary A-V fistula	Blood loss may be impossible to control. IV may be difficult to maintain due to poor tissues. More than 90 percent have recurrent chest infection, dyspnea, cyanosis, clubbing by age 60
Osteogenesis imperfecta (fragilitas ossium)	I. Congenita - stillborn and rapidly fatal. II. Tarda - Pathological fractures. Osteoporosis leads to kyphoscoliosis	Chest deformity leads to lung pathology. Fragile vessels lead to subcutaneous hemorrhage. Dentin deficiency causes caries and easily broken teeth. Extreme care in positioning
Patau syndrome (trisomy 13)	Mental retardation 100 percent. Microcephaly, micrognathia and/or dextrocardia. Cleft lip or palate. Congenital heart disease. Usually fatal by three years	Difficult intubation. Usually VSD.

Pendred syndrome	Deafness and goiter. Incomplete block of thyroxine production	May be euthyroid or hypothyroid. Make sure euthyroid pre-op. Otherwise as for cretinism
Phenylketonuria	Phenylalanine hydroxylase deficiency. Vomiting, irritability, mental retardation. Hypertonia, convulsions. Very sensitive to narcotics and other CNS depressants	Inhalation induction and maintenance. Continue anti-epileptic drugs. Tendency to hypoglycemia - 100 percent. Require dextrose infusion
Pierre Robin syndrome	Cleft palate, micrognathia, glossoptosis. Associated congenital heart disease may occur	Newborn may asphyxiate - nurse prone on frame. May require tongue suture, intubation or tracheostomy. May be very difficult to intubate. Awake intubation
Polycystic kidneys	One-third have associated cysts in liver, pancreas, spleen, lungs, bladder, thyroid. Cerebral aneurysm in 15 percent	Care with renally excreted drugs. Beware lung cysts: may lead to pneumothorax. Avoid hypertension because of possible cerebral aneurysm
Polysplenia	Bilateral visceral left sidedness (see also asplenia - converse)	Complex cardiac anomalies common: ASD and endocardial cushion defects. Usually not so complex as in asplenia
Pompe's disease (glycogen storage II)	Muscle deposits - severe hypotonicity. Massive cardiomegaly. Death before two years of age	Extreme care, avoidance respiratory depressants, muscle relaxants, cardiac depressants. Large tongue may cause airway problem

Name	***Description***	***Anesthetic Implications***
Porphyria	Paralysis, psychiatric disorder. Autonomic imbalance - hypertension, tachycardia. Abdominal pain precipitated by drugs, infections, etc.	*Avoid* barbiturates including thiopental. Sedatives - meprobamate, Librium, glutethimide, carbromal. Hydroxydione (steroid anesthetic). Nikethamide. Hydantoin derivatives. Sulfonamides. Antipyretics. Hypoglycemic agents. *Have been used safely*: chlorpromazine, promazine, promethazine, chloral, propanidid, morphine, pethidine. Procaine. N20. Ether. Succinylcholine, 4-tubocurarine, gallamine. Atropine and neostigmine. Pentolinium
Prader-Willi syndrome	*Neonate* - hypotonia, poor feeding, absent reflexes. *Second phase* - hyperactive, uncontrollable polyphagia, mental retardation	Obesity of extreme proportions leading to cardio-pulmonary failure
Prune Belly syndrome	Agenesis of abdominal musculature with renal anomalies	Poor cough - respiratory infections. Respiration requires use of accessory muscles. Treat as full stomach. Intubate and assist or control ventilation. Avoid muscle relaxants. Beware possible renal failure
Pyle's disease (metaphyseal dysplasia)	Craniofacial abnormalities. Enlarged mandible. Cranial N. paralyses	No described anesthetic problem

Rieger syndrome	Myotonic dystrophy and other myopathies. Hypoplasia of maxilla, abnormal teeth, mental retardation. Occasional imperforate anus	Anesthetic requirements dictated by associated muscle disease - see myotonia congenita, myotonic dystrophy
Riley-Day syndrome (familial dysautonomia)	Deficiency of dopamine hydroxylase. Hyper- and hypotensive attacks, absent lacrimation, abnormal sweating. Insensitive to pain. Poor suckling and swallowing	Emotional lability. Recurrent aspiration, pneumonia and chronic lung disease. Labile blood pressure - care with halothane, etc. Sensitive to adrenergic and cholinergic drugs. Pre-medication - atropine and chlorpromazine. Respiratory center insensitive to CO_2 - need IPPV. Avoid respiratory depressants
Rubinstein syndrome	Mental retardation, microcephaly. Frequent chest infections. Swallowing abnormality. Congenital heart disease	Repeated aspiration leads to pneumonia and chronic lung disease
Scheie disease (mucopolysaccharidosis V)	Corneal clouding, hernias. Joint stiffness especially hands and feet. Aortic valve involvement	Aortic incompetence by third decade. Joint stiffness - care in positioning
Scleroderma	Diffuse cutaneous stiffening. Plastic surgery required for contractures and constrictions	Scarring face and mouth - difficult airway and intubation. Chest restriction - poor compliance. Diffuse pulmonary fibrosis - hypoxia. Veins - often invisible and impalpable. Cardiac fibrosis or cor pulmonale. History of steroid therapy

Name	Description	Anesthetic Implications
Sebaceous nevi (linear)	Linear nevi from forehead to nose. Hydrocephalus, mental retardation, associated with coarctation and hypoplasia of aorta	Cardiovascular complications
Shy-Drager syndrome	Orthostatic hypotension. Diffuse degeneration of central and autonomic nervous systems. Decreased sweating. Hypersensitive to angiotensin and epinephrine	Labile pulse and blood pressure possibly due to defective baroreceptor response - avoid methoxyflurane, cyclopropane and ether. Cautious use of halothane. Treat hypotension with infusion phenylephrine
Silver syndrome	Short stature, skeletal asymmetry. Micrognathia. Abnormal sexual development	Possibly difficult intubation
Smith-Lemli-Opitz syndrome	Mental retardation. Genital and skeletal anomalies - micrognathia. Thymic hypoplasia	Airway and intubation problems. Pneumonia, possible increased susceptibility to infection
Sotos syndrome (cerebral gigantism)	Acromegalic features. Dilated ventricles but normal intracranial pressure	All features non-progressive. Possible airway problems due to acromegalic skull. No other described problems

Stevens-Johnson syndrome	Erythema multiforme, urticarial lesions and erosions of mouth, eyes and genitalia. Possibly hypersensitivity to exogenous agents, i.e., drugs.	Oral lesions - avoid intubation and esophageal stethoscope. Monitoring difficult because of skin lesions but essential. ECG - fibrillation, myocarditis, pericarditis occur. Temperature control - febrile episodes. Intravenous infusion - essential but avoid cut-down, because of infection. Ketamine probably best anesthetic. Pleural blebs and pneumothorax may occur
Sturge-Weber syndrome	Cavernous angioma over trigeminal nerve, 1-3 divisions. Intracranial calcification, convulsions and maybe progressive neurological deficits	No specific anesthetic problems
Supravalvular aortic stenosis syndrome (idiopathic infantile hypercalcemia) (William's syndrome)	Hypercalcemia and mental retardation. Abnormal facies. Cardiac - dyspnea, angina. Therapy, low calcium diet, steroids. Cardiac surgery	Fixed cardiac output and ischemia. History of steroids. Monitor serum Ca^{++}
Tay-Sach's disease	Gangliosidosis. Blindness and progressive dementia and degeneration of central nervous system	No described anesthetic hazard. Progressive neurological loss leads to respiratory complications. Supportive measures only treatment
Thomsen's disease	See Myotonia congenita	

Name	Description	Anesthetic Implications
Thrombocytopenia with absent radius	Episodic thrombocytopenia precipitated by stress, infection, surgery, etc. Low platelets improve to normal by adulthood. Congenital heart disease in 30 percent.	Platelet transfusion for surgery or bleeding (35-40 percent die in first year of intracranial hemorrhage). Avoid elective surgery in first year
Treacher Collins syndrome (mandibulo-facial dysostosis)	Micrognathia and aplastic zygomatic arches. Microstomia, choanal atresia. Congenital heart disease may occur	Possible airway and intubation difficulties. Less severe than Pierre Robin deformity
Tuberous sclerosis	Adenoma sebaceum of skin, epilepsy and mental retardation. Intracranial calcification in 50 percent. Hamartomas in lungs, kidneys, heart	Kidneys - pyelonephritis and renal failure. Care with renally excreted drugs. Lungs - possible rupture of lung cysts. Possible cardiac arrhythmia
Turner's syndrome	XO chromosome. Micrognathia, coarctation, dissecting aneurysm of aorta or pulmonary stenosis. Renal anomalies in more than 50 percent	Possibly difficult intubation. Cardiovascular abnormality. Possible renal disease - care with renally excreted drugs
Von Gierke's disease	Glycogen storage disease I. Hepatomegaly, enlarged kidneys, severe attacks of hypoglycemia	Monitor blood sugar and acid-base balance (IV glucose infusion). Diazoxide for hypoglycemia
von-Hippel-Lindau syndrome	Retinal or CNS hemangioblastoma. (Posterior fossa or spinal cord). Associated with pheochromocytoma, renal, pancreatic, or hepatic cysts	Problems due to associated pheochromocytoma, renal and hepatic pathology

von-Recklinghausen disease (neurofibromatosis)	Cafe-au-lait spots. Tumors all parts CNS. Peripheral tumors associated with nerve trunks. Increased incidence pheochromocytoma. Fifty percent kyphoscoliosis. Honeycomb cystic lung changes. Renal artery dysplasia and hypertension	Screen for pheochromocytoma (urinary VMA). Should be investigated for lung function. Tumors may occur in the larynx and right ventricle outflow tract. Care with renally excreted drugs if kidneys involved
von Willebrand's disease (pseudohemophilia)	Prolonged bleeding time (decreased factor VIII activity) due to defective platelet adhesiveness. ? Capillary abnormality	Bleeding can be controlled by fresh or fresh frozen plasma, cryoprecipitate. Avoid salicylate therapy (effect on platelets, possible GI bleeding)
Weber Christian disease (chronic non-suppurative panniculitis)	Necrosis of fat, any location including retroperitoneal, pericardial, meningeal	Involvement of retroperitoneal tissues may cause acute or chronic adrenal insufficiency, of pericardium leads to restrictive pericarditis, of meninges causes convulsions. Avoid trauma to fat by heat, cold or pressure
Werdig-Hoffman disease	Infantile muscular atrophy more severe than Welander. Feeding difficulties, aspiration, usually death before puberty	Chronic respiratory problems. Minimal anesthesia required. Avoid muscle relaxants and respiratory depressant drugs. Ventilatory support may be required and weaning may be difficult

Name	Description	Anesthetic Implications
Werner syndrome	Premature aging, diabetes. Early cataracts. Mental retardation in 50 percent. Bony lesions like osteomyelitis. Cardiac infarction and failure	Anesthesia as for adult with myocardial ischemia
Wermer syndrome (multiple endocrine adenomatosis type I)	Hyperparathyroidism. Tumors of pituitary and pancreatic islet cells. Gastric ulcer. Occasionally have carcinoid tumors of bronchial tree	Renal failure due to stones. Hypoglycemia secondary to hyperinsulinism
Wilson's disease (hepatolenticular degeneration)	Decreased ceruloplasmin causes abnormal copper deposits especially in liver and CNS motor nuclei. Renal tubular acidosis	Hepatic failure due to fibrosis. Thiopental may be used in small doses. Muscle relaxants - succinylcholine apnea rare despite pseudocholinesterase reduction. d-tubocurarine - short action due to globin binding. Care with renally excreted drugs
Wilson-Mikity syndrome	Prematurity < 1500 gm birth weight. Severe chronic lung disease leading to fibrosis and cystic areas etiology - ? oxygen toxicity	Right heart failure. Repeated chest infection and aspiration. Use of steroids to prevent pulmonary fibrosis

Wolff-Parkinson-White syndrome	ECG abnormality - Short P.R., prolonged QRS with phasic variation in 40 percent. Associated with many cardiac defects. Anomalous conduction path between atria and ventricles. Delta wave may be present on ECG	Scopolamine preferred to atropine as drying agent. Tachycardia due to atropine or apprehension may change ECG and suggest infarction, with ST segment depression. Paroxysmal SVT on induction of anesthesia or during cardiac surgery has been reported. Should be treated with digitalis, propranolol, pacemaker if necessary. Neostigmine may accentuate W-P-W pattern
Wolfman's disease (familial xanthomatosis)	Adrenal calcification. Resembles Niemann-Pick disease with hepatosplenomegaly and hypersplenism. Involvement other tissues from foam cells, including myocardium	Anemia, thrombocytopenia. Platelet transfusion only successful post-splenectomy

Cross Index of Alternative Names

Acrocephalosyndactyly - Apert syndrome
Albinism - Chediak-Higashi syndrome, Hermansky syndrome
Amaurosis congenita - Leber syndrome
Anhidrotic ectodermal dysplasia - Christ-Siemens-Touraine
Bournville's disease - Tuberous sclerosis
Branched chain ketonuria - Maple-Syrup urine disease
Cardio-Auditory syndrome - Jervell-Nielson syndrome
Cerebrohepatorenal syndrome - Bowens syndrome
Chondrodystrophies - Conradi syndrome, Ellis-van-Creveld syndrome
Connective tissue disorders - Cutis Laxa, Ehlers Danlos syndrome, Groenblad-Strandberg syndrome, Marfan's syndrome
Cranial synostoses - Apert syndrome, Carpenters syndrome, Chotzen syndrome, Crouzon syndrome, Noack syndrome
Enchondromatoses - Maffucci syndrome, Olliers syndrome
Eulenberg disease - Paramyotonia congenita
Familial dysautonomia - Riley Day syndrome
Fragilitas Ossium - Osteogenesis imperfecta
Glycogen Storage Diseases - I Von Gierke, II Pompe, III Forbes, IV Anderson, V McArdle, VI Hers, VII Lewis
Goiter - Cretinism, Pendred's syndrome
Heart and Hand syndrome - Hold-Oram syndrome
Heredity hemorrhagic telangiectasia - Osler-Weber-Rendu syndrome
Hepatolenticular degeneration - Wilson's disease
Histiocytosis X Syndromes - Hand Schuller-Christian, Letterer-Siew, Urbach-Wiethe
Homogentisic-Aciduria - Alkaptonuria
Hutchinson-Gilford syndrome - Progeria
Idiopathic Infantile Hypercalcemia - see supravalvular aortic stenosis syndrome
Immunodeficiency Syndromes - Ataxia telangiectasia, Chediak-Higashi, Chronic granulomatous disease, Wiskott-Aldrich syndrome
Lipid storage diseases - Fabry's disease, Gauchers disease, Niemann-Pick disease, Tay-Sacks disease, Wolman's disease
Lipogranulomatosis - Farber's disease

Louis-Bar disease - Ataxia Telangiectasia
Mandibulo-Facial dysostosis - Treacher-Collins syndrome
Marble-bone disease - Albers Schonberg
Mongolism - Down's syndrome
Mucopolysaccharidoses - I Hurler, II Hunter, III San Filippo, IV Morquio-Ullrich, V Scheie, VI Maroteaux-Lamy
Multiple Endocrine Adenomatoses - I Wermer Syndrome, II Sipple Syndrome
Muscular atrophy - myotonia congenita, Welanders muscular atrophy, Werdnig-Hoffman disease
Muscular dystrophy - Duchenne, Central core (Shy Magee), Reigers syndrome
Myotonic syndromes - myotonia congenita, dystrophia myotonica, Reigers syndrome
Neonatal hypoglycemia - Beckwith syndrome, Idiopathic, Glycogen-storage disease esp. Pompe's
Oculoauriculovertebral syndrome - Goldenhar syndrome
Oculocerebrorenal syndrome - Lowe syndrome
Pheochromocytoma - Sipple syndrome, von-Hippel-Lindau syndrome, von Recklinghausen syndrome
Pseudohypoparathyroidism - Albright's Osteodystrophy
Renal Tubular Acidosis - Albright Butler syndrome, Fanconi syndrome, Lowes syndrome
Shy-Magee - Central core disease
Total lipoatrophy - Lipodystrophy
Telangiectasia - Ataxia telangiectasis, Osler-Weber-Rendu syndrome
Thrombasthenia - Glanzmann's disease
Thrombotic thrombocytopenic purpura - Moschkowitz disease

Adapted with permission from reference 76.

Obstetric Anesthesia

Summary of Ventilatory Changes during Pregnancy

Parameters	Normal Non-pregnant Non-Female	Gravida at Term	Change*
Tidal volume in ml	450	650	+45%
Respiratory rate per minute	15	16	+10%
Minute ventilation in liters	6.5	10	+55%
Inspiratory capacity (IC) in liters	2.5	2.75	+10%
Expiratory reserve volume (ERV) in liters	0.7	0.55	-20%
Residual volume (RV) in liters	1.0	0.8	-20%
Functional residual capacity (FRC) in liters	1.7	1.35	-20%
Vital capacity (VC) in liters	3.2	3.2	None
Timed vital capacity			
a. 1 second	82%	80%	Insignificant
b. 2 seconds	93%	94%	Insignificant
c. 3 seconds	98%	98%	None
Maximum breathing capacity (MBC) in liters	102	97	-5%
Total lung volume in liters	4.2	4.1	-5%
Maximum air flows in liters per minute			
a. Inspiratory	150	135	- 13%
b. Expiratory	100	98	-2%
Airway resistance in cm H_2O/liter/second	2.5	2.5	None
Walking ventilation in liters per minute	15	19	+30%
Walking dyspnea index—%	15	21	+40%

*Calculated in round figures.

Reproduced with permission from reference 78.

Pulmonary volumes and capacities in the nonpregnant state

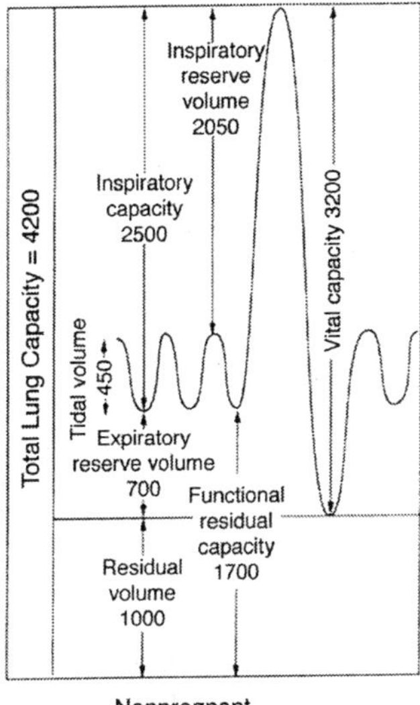

Nonpregnant

Reprinted with permission from reference 78.

Pulmonary volumes and capacities in the gravida at term

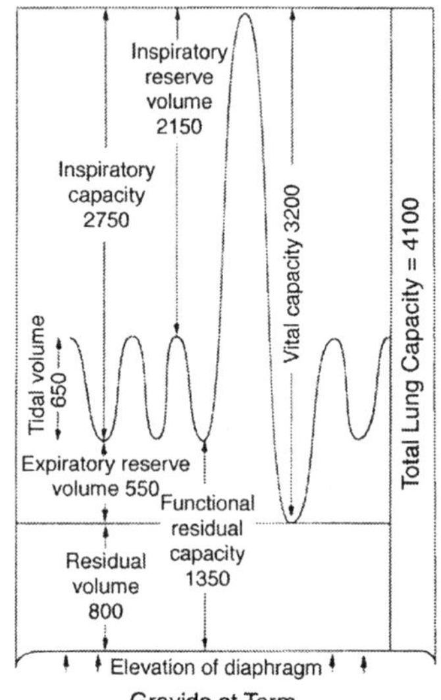

Reprinted with permission from reference 78.

Changes in the Cardiovascular System with Pregnancy

Variable	Direction of Change	Average Change (%)
Blood volume	↑	+35
Plasma volume	↑	+45
Red blood cell volume	↑	+20
Cardiac output	↑	+40
Stroke volume	↑	+30
Heart rate	↑	+15
Femoral (uterine) venous pressure	↑	+ 15 mmHg
Total peripheral resistance	↓	- 15
Mean arterial blood pressure	↓	- 15 mmHg
Systolic blood pressure	↓	- 0 - 15 mmHg
Diastolic blood pressure	↓	- 10 - 20 mmHg
Central venous pressure	±	no change

Reproduced with permission from reference 77.

Changes in Gastrointestinal Physiology During Pregnany*

Parameter	Trimester			Labor	Postpartum (1-3 hr)
	First	Second	Third		
Barrier pressure#	Decreased	Decreased	Decreased	Decreased	?
Gastric emptying	No change	No change	No change	Decreased	No change
Gastric acid secretion	Decreased	Decreased	No change	?	?
Proportion of women with gastric volume > 25 mL	No change	No change	No change	Increased	No change
Proportion of women with gastric pH < 2.5	No change	No change	No change	Decreased	No change

*Relative to nonpregnant women.
#Difference between intragastric pressure and tone of the lower esophageal high pressure zone.

Reproduced with permission from reference 79.

Changes in Blood and Its Constituents During Pregnancy Average Values

Variable	Nonpregnant	Term Pregnancy	Change
A. Volumes (ml)			
Total blood	4000	5800	+45%
Plasma	2700	4200	+55%
Red cell	1400	2800	+30%
B. Formed Elements			
RBC (million/mm^3)	4.6	4.3*	-0.3
Hemoglobin (g/dl)	14	12.8*	-1.2
Hematocrit (%)	41	36.5	-4.5
WBC	6,000	9,000	+ 3,000
Platelets	300,000	260,000	- 40,000
C. Total Proteins			
Amount (gm)	290	390	↑
Concentration (gm/100 ml)	7.3	6.5	↓
D. Albumin			
Total (gm)	127	144	↑
Concentration (gm/100 ml)	5.5	4.4	↓
E. Total Globulins		Slight relative and absolute increase	
Alpha		Slight increase	
Beta		Slight increase	
Gamma		Slight increase	

Variable	Nonpregnant	Term Pregnancy	Change
F. Electrolytes (mEq/L)			
Total Base	155	148	↓
Na^+	143	138	↓
K^-	4.3	4.1	↓
Ca^{++}	4.4	4.6	↑
Cl^-	105	103	↓
Mg^{++}	1.67	1.52	↓
HPO^-	1.96	1.15	↓
$HC0_{3-}$	26	21-23	↓
G. Blood Gases and Acid-Base			
PaO_2 (mm Hg)	95	105	↑
$PaCO_2$ (mm Hg)	40	30	↓
Buffer base (mEq/L)	47	42	↓
Base excess (mEq/L)	0.0	- 1.5	↓
pH	7.40	7.44	slight ↑

* Values at term after iron and folic acid supplementation.

Reproduced with permission from reference 78.

Effects Of Pregnancy And Of Estrogen Administration On Tests Used To Evaluate Thyroid Function

Tests	Normal Pregnancy	Estrogen Administration	Hyperthyroidism
Basal Metabolic Rate	Increased	Not Increased	Increased
Total Thyroxine	Increased	Increased	Increased
Thyroxine-Binding Globulin	Increased	Increased	Not Increased
Free Thyroxine	Not Increased	Not Increased	Increased
Total Triiodothyronine	Increased	Increased	Increased
Free Triiodothyronine	Not Increased	Not Increased	Increased
Radioiodine Uptake (Percent)	Increased	Not Increased	Increased
Absolute Iodine Uptake	Not Increased	Not Increased	Increased
Triiodothyronine Resin Uptake	Decreased	Decreased	Increased
Serum Cholesterol Level	Increased	Variable	Decreased

Reproduced with permission from reference 80.

Indicators Of Severity Of Pregnancy-Induced Hypertension

Abnormality	Mild	Severe
Diastolic Blood Pressure	< 100 mm Hg	≥ 110 mm Hg
Proteinuria	Trace to 1+	Persistent 2+ or more
Headache	Absent	Present
Visual Disturbances	Absent	Present
Upper Abdominal Pain	Absent	Present
Oliguria	Absent	Present
Convulsions	Absent	Present
Serum Creatinine	Normal	Elevated
Thrombocytopenia	Absent	Present
Hyperbilirubinemia	Absent	Present
SGOT Elevation	Minimal	Marked
Fetal Growth Retardation	Absent	Obvious

Reproduced with permission from reference 80.

Diagnosis of Preeclampsia and HELLP Syndrome

Preeclampsia	**HEELP Syndrome** (H for hemolysis, EL for elevated liver function tests, and LP for low platelet count)
1. Blood Pressure ≥ 160/110 mmHg	1. Hemolysis, defined by abnormal peripheral smear, increased bilirubin (≥ 1.2 mg/dl), and increased lactate dehydrogenase (> 600 U/L).
2. Proteinuria ≥ 5 g/24 h	2. Elevated liver enzymes, defined as increased SGOT (> 70 U/L) and increased LDH
3. Oliguria < 400 ml/24 h	3. Thrombocytopenia (< 100,000)
4. Neurological disturbances	
5. Pulmonary edema	

Indications for Pulmonary Artery Catheter Placement in the Severe Preeclamptic or Eclamptic Patient: Findings and Their Therapy

1. Unresponsive or refractory hypertension
   a. Increased systemic vascular resistance (Rx: vasodilators)
   b. Increased cardiac output (Rx: decrease preload with nitroglycerin or decrease cardiac output with a β-blocker)
2. Pulmonary edema
   a. Cardiogenic or left ventricular failure (Rx: afterload reduction or inotropes)
   b. Increased systemic vascular resistance (Rx: afterload reduction)
   c. Noncardiogenic volume overload (Rx: diuretics, fluid restriction)
   d. Decreased colloid oncotic pressure (Rx: 25% albumin, fluid restriction)
3. Persistent arterial desaturation; unable to distinguish between cardiac and noncardiac origin
4. Oliguria unresponsive to modest fluid loading
   a. Low preload (Rx: crystalloid infusion)
   b. Severe increased systemic vascular resistance with low cardiac output (Rx: afterload reduction)
   c. Selective renal artery vasoconstriction

Adapted with permission from reference 81.

Various Actions of Magnesium Sulfate as Used in Preeclampsia-Eclampsia

Beneficial effects for preeclampsia-eclampsia	Detrimental effects
1. Anticonvulsant	1. Tocolysis with prolonged labor and increased postpartum hemorrhage
2. Vasodilation	2. Decreased fetal heart rate variability
Increased uterine blood flow	3. Myoneural blocking effects
Increased renal blood flow	Generalized muscle weakness
Antihypertensive (unreliable)	Increased sensitivity to muscle relaxants, especially nondepolarizing muscle relaxants
3. Increased prostacyclin release by endothelial cells	4. Neonatal effects: lower Apgar scores and decreased muscle ton (only with maternal overdose)
4. Decreased plasma renin activity	
5. Decreased angiotensin-converting enzyme	
6. Attenuation of vascular responses to pressor substances	
7. Reduced platelet aggregation	
8. Bronchodilation	
9. Tocolysis: improves uterine blood flow and antagonizes uterine hyperactivity	

Reproduced with permission from reference 82.

Effects of Increasing Plasma Magnesium Levels

Plasma Mg (mEq/liter)	Effects
1.5 - 2	Normal plasma level
4 - 8	Therapeutic range (for preeclampsia/ eclampsia/convulsions)
5 - 10	Electrocardiographic changes P-R interval prolonged QRS complex widening
10	Loss of deep tendon reflexes
15	Respiratory paralysis
15	Sinoatrial and atrioventricular block
25	Cardiac arrest

Reproduced with permission from reference 83.

Note: Treatment of a magnesium overdose consists of support of ventilation and intravenous administration of a calcium salt to antagonize the effects of magnesium. Hemodialysis and peritoneal dialysis are also effective.

Side Effects of Tocolytics

Drug	Maternal Effects	Fetal Effects
Beta-adrenergic agents	↓ Blood pressure ↑ Heart rate Congestive heart failure Dysrhythmias Pulmonary edema Headache ↑ Glucose ↓ Potassium	↑ Heart rate ↑ Glucose
Magnesium sulfate	Pulmonary edema Drowsiness ↑ Sensitivity to muscle relaxants	Hypotonia
Calcium channel blockers	↓ Blood pressure ↓ Cardiac conduction	

Reproduced with permission from reference 84.

The Friedman Curve

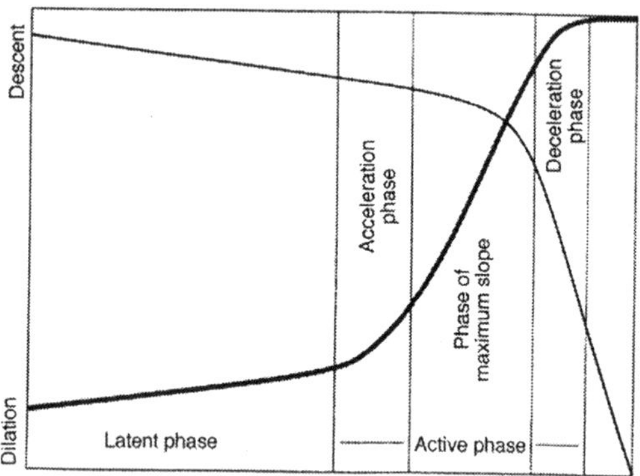

Reproduced with permission from reference 86.

Labor length

Stage of labor	Mean	Median	Mode	Limit
Nulliparous				
First stage (hr)	14.4	12.3	9.5	-
Latent phase (hr)	8.6	7.5	6.0	<u>20</u>
Active phase (hr)	4.9	4.0	3.0	12
Maximum slope (cm/hr)	3.0	2.7	1.5	<u>1.2</u>
Second stage (hr)	I.0	0.8	0.6	2.5
Parous				
First stage (hr)	7.7	6.5	5.1	-
Latent phase (hr)	5.3	4.5	3.5	<u>14</u>
Active phase (hr)	2.2	1.8	1.5	5.2
Maximum slope	5.7	5.2	4.5	<u>1.5</u>
Second stage (hr)	0.2	0.2	0.1	0.8

Important limits are underlined.

Modified with permission from reference 87.

Usual Indications for Cesarean Section

I. Fetopelvic disproportion
- A. Pelvic (the Passage) insufficiency
  - 1. Bony pelvis
    - a. Pelvic inlet (usually anterior-posterior <10 cm)
    - b. Midpelvis (usually transverse, ie, ischial spines <9.5 cm)
    - c. Outlet (very unusual and then almost never seen in the absence of other pelvic contractures)
  - 2. Soft tissue obstruction
    - a. Low lying placenta (especially posteriorly implanted)
    - b. Uterine leiomyomata
    - c. Ovarian tumors
    - d. Other genital tract neoplasia (rare)
- B. Fetal complications (the Passenger)
  - 1. Normal fetus
    - a. Macrosomia (>4,000 g)
    - b. Malposition and malpresentation
      - i. Breech unfavorable for vaginal delivery
      - ii. Deflexed head
      - iii. Transverse or oblique lie
      - iv. Brow
      - v. Posterior mental position
      - vi. Shoulder presentations
      - vii. Compound presentations
  - 2. Anomalous fetus
    - a. Meningomyelocele
    - b. Hydrocephalus
    - c. Sacrococcygeal teratoma
    - d. Miscellaneous fetal anomalies
  - 3. Multiple gestation
    - a. Twins
      - i. Twin A any presentation except vertex
      - ii. Twin B not suitable for vaginal delivery
      - iii. Failure of intrapartum external version
      - iv. Fetal distress (even if Twin A has been delivered vaginally)
      - v. All monoamniotic twins
    - b. Triplets or greater number
- C. Abnormalities of the labor (the Powers)
  - 1. Primary uterine inertia
    - a. Prolonged latent phase (unusual, but >20 hr in a nullipara and >14 hr in a multipara)
    - b. Protraction disorders
      - i. Protracted active phase dilatation (nulligravida >1.2 cm/hr multigravida >1.5 cm/hr)
      - ii. Protracted descent (nulligravida > 1 cm/hr, multigravida >2 cm/hr)

        c. Arrest disorders
            i. Prolonged deceleration phase (nulliparas ~3 h, multiparas ~1 h)
            ii. Secondary arrest of dilatation (no dilation for ~2 h)
            iii. Active phase arrest of descent (~1 h)
            iv. Failure of descent in the deceleration phase or second stage (~1 h)
    2. Uterine inertia due to fetopelvic disproportion
    3. Failed induction

II. Fetal distress
  A. Uteroplacental insufficiency
  B. Cord accidents
  C. Metabolic acidosis

III. Obstetric hemorrhage (maternal and/or fetal)
  A. Abruptio placenta
  B. Placenta previa
  C. Ruptured uterus
  D. Vasa previa

IV. Infections
  A. Severe chorioamnionitis
  B. Active maternal genital herpes
  C. Active maternal condylomata acuminata

V. Maternal and/or fetal complications potentially adversely influenced by labor and/or vaginal delivery
  A. Antepartal testing indicative of labor intolerance
  B. Cervical dystocia
  C. Medical
    1. Fulminating preeclampsia-eclampsia
    2. Diabetes
    3. Erythroblastosis
    4. Severe maternal heart disease
    5. Other debilitating conditions
  D. Surgical
    1. Cervical or uterine scarring of extent that may rupture with labor (e.g., extensive myomectomy, trachelorrhaphy)
    2. Cervical cerclage
        a. All abdominal cervical cerclages
        b. Certain vaginal cerclages (e.g., cannot remove)
    3. Serious maternal problems (e.g., vesicovaginal or rectovaginal fistula)
    4. Prior extensive vaginal plastic operations
    5. Carcinoma of the cervix

VI. Repeat cesarean

Reprinted with permission from reference 88.

Categories of Emergency Cesarean Section

Examples	Preferred anesthetic
Stable	
Chronic uteroplacental insufficiency Abnormal fetal presentation with ruptured membranes (not in labor)	Epidural, spinal
Urgent	
Dystocia Failed trial of forceps Active genital herpes infection with rupture of membranes Previous classic cesarean section and active labor Cord prolapse without fetal distress Variable decelerations with prompt recovery and normal FHR variability	Extension of preexisting epidural anesthesia or spinal
Stat	
Massive maternal hemorrhage Ruptured uterus Cord prolapse with fetal bradycardia Agonal fetal distress (e.g., prolonged bradycardia or late decelerations with no FHR variability)	General unless there is adequate preexisting epidural anesthesia

Modified with permission from reference 89.

Treatment of the Fetus in Utero

Events Inciting Abnormal Pattern	Possible FHR Patterns	Corrective Maneuver	Mechanism
Hypotension (e.g., supine hypotension, conduction anesthesia)	Bradycardia; late decelerations	Intravenous fluids, position change, ephedrine	Restoration of uterine blood flow toward normal
Excessive uterine activity	Bradycardia; late decelerations	Decrease in oxytocin; lateral position	Restoration of uterine blood flow toward normal
Transient umbilical cord compression	Variable decelerations	Change in maternal position (e.g., left or right lateral, Trendelenburg)	Restoration of umbilical blood flow toward normal
Head compression in second stage	Early decelerations	Discourage "pushing" efforts; change in maternal position (e.g., left or right lateral, Trendelenburg)	Restoration of umbilical blood flow toward normal
Decreased uterine blood flow (below limits of fetal basal O_2 needs) associated with uterine contraction	Late decelerations	Change in maternal position (e.g., left lateral, Trendelenburg); establishment of maternal hyperoxia (?Tocolytic agents, e.g., ritodrine or terbutaline)	Enhancement of uterine blood flow to optimum; increase in maternal-fetal O_2 gradient (Decrease in contractions, thus abolishing associated decrease of uterine blood flow)
Prolonged asphyxia	Decreasing FHR variability	Change in maternal position (e.g., left lateral, Trendelenburg); establishment of maternal hyperoxia	Enhancement of uterine blood flow to optimum; increase in maternal-fetal O_2 gradient

Reproduced with permission from reference 85.

Rapid Estimation of Gestational Age of the Newborn

Sites	Gestational Age		
	36 Weeks Or Less	**37 to 38 Weeks**	**39 Weeks or More**
Sole Creases	Anterior transverse crease only	Occasional creases anterior two-thirds	Sole covered with creases
Breast Nodule Diameter	2 mm	4 mm	7 mm
Scalp Hair	Fine and fuzzy	Fine and fuzzy	Coarse and silky
Ear Lobe	Pliable, no cartilage	Some cartilage	Stiffened by thick cartilage
Testes and Scrotum	Testes in lower canal, scrotum small, few rugae	Intermediate	Testes pendulous, scrotum full, extensive rugae

Reproduced with permission from reference 80.

Normal Values for Oxygen, Carbon Dioxide, and pH in Human Maternal and Fetal Blood

	Uterine		Umbilical	
	Artery	Vein	Vein	Artery
PO_2 (mm Hg)	95	40	27	15
O_2Hb (percent saturation)	98	76	68	30
O_2 Content (ml/dl)	15.8	12.2	14.5	6.4
Hemoglobin (gm/dl)	12.0	12.0	16.0	16.0
O_2 Capacity (ml O_2/dl)	16.1	16.1	21.4	21.4
PCO_2 (mm Hg)	32	40	43	48
CO_2 Content (mM/L)	19.6	21.8	25.2	26.3
HCO_3 (mEq/L)	18.8	20.7	24.0	25.0
pH	7.40	7.34	7.38	7.35

Reproduced with permission from reference 80.

Steps to Minimize Pulmonary Aspiration in the Obstetric Patient

1. Allow actively laboring patients only ice chips or small sips of water per os. Those patients at particular risk of an operative delivery should only receive sufficient quantities to keep them comfortable, and ideally should be kept NPO.
2. Carefully evaluate airway of all patients admitted to Labor Suite.
3. Avoid oversedation.
4. Utilize regional anesthesia and avoid general anesthesia whenever possible.
5. Preface any anesthetic or obstetric intervention (e.g., immediately prior to initiation of epidural analgesia, or shortly before vaginal delivery) with 15 - 30 ml 0.3M sodium citrate solution or Bicitra. - *(Note, this is thought to be optional by some practitioners.)*
6. Avoid hypotension, aortocaval compression, local anesthetic toxicity, and excessively high blocks.
7. In patients recognized as being at particular risk, (e.g., the morbidly obese patient), consider use of ranitidine **and** metoclopramide.
8. Should general anesthesia become necessary use a rapid-sequence intubation technique with cricoid pressure properly maintained until the endotracheal tube cuff has been inflated and end-tidal CO_2 sensed. Ideally an experienced anesthesiologist should be in attendance.
9. Educate all members of the obstetric team on a "failed intubation drill."
10. On emergence from general anesthesia, extubate only when the patient is fully responsive with no evidence of residual neuromuscular blockade.
11. Provide appropriate continuous observation of all obstetric patients during labor, delivery, and the immediate postpartum period.

Reproduced with permission from reference 90.

General Anesthesia: Anesthetic Implications of Maternal Physiologic Changes

Endotracheal intubation

- Smaller endotracheal tubes required
- Increased risk of trauma with nasotracheal intubation
- Increased risk of failed intubation

Maternal oxygenation

- Increased physiologic shunt when supine
- Increased rate of denitrogenation
- Increased rate of decline of PaO_2 during apnea

Maternal ventilation

- Increased minute ventilation required

Adapted with permission from reference 91.

Regional Anesthesia: Anesthetic Implications of Maternal Physiologic Changes

Technical considerations

- Lumbar lordosis increased
- Head-down tilt when in lateral position
- CSF return unaltered
- Reduced sensitivity of "hanging drop" technique

Hydration

- Increased fluid requirements to prevent hypotension*

Local anesthetic dose requirements#

- Subarachnoid dose reduced 20% to 33%
- Epidural dose (large dose) unaltered
- Epidural dose (small dose) reduced

* Relative to that required by nonpregnant women.
# Change in the segmental dose requirement relative to nonpregnant women.

Adapted with permission from reference 91.

General Anesthesia: Pharmacology During Pregnancy

Inhalation anesthetics

- Minimum alveolar concentration reduced 20% to 40%
- Rate of induction increased

Induction agents

- ED_{50} of thiopental reduced 35%
- Elimination half-life of thiopental prolonged
- Elimination half-life of propofol unaltered

Meperidine

- Elimination half-life unaltered

Succinylcholine

- Duration of blockade unaltered (or decreased)
- Sensitivity reduced

Nondepolarizing muscle relaxants

- ED_{50} of vecuronium reduced
- Elimination half-life of vecuronium and pancuronium shortened
- Duration of blockade of atracurium unaltered

Chronotropic agents

- Response diminished

Pressors

- Response variable

*Changes relative to nonpregnant women.

Reprinted with permission from reference 91.

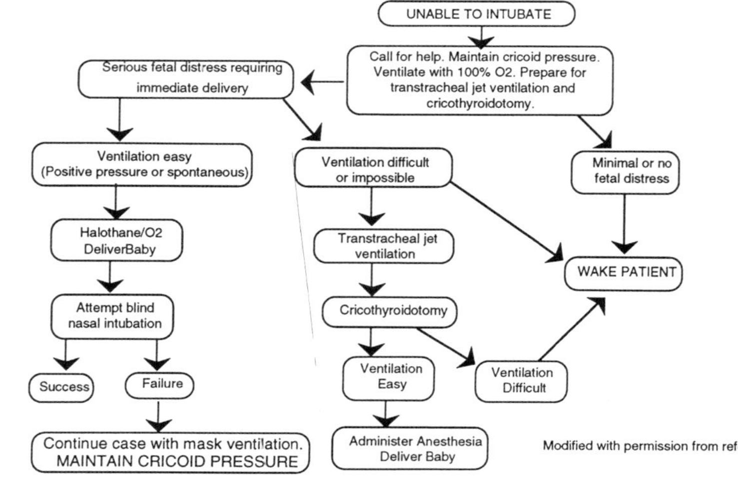
Algorithm for Management of the Difficult Obstetric Intubation
UNABLE TO INTUBATE
Call for help. Maintain cricoid pressure. Ventilate with 100% O2. Prepare for transtracheal jet ventilation and cricothyroidotomy.
Serious fetal distress requiring immediate delivery
Minimal or no fetal distress
Ventilation easy (Positive pressure or spontaneous)
Ventilation difficult or impossible
WAKE PATIENT
Halothane/O2 DeliverBaby
Transtracheal jet ventilation
Attempt blind nasal intubation
Cricothyroidotomy
Success
Failure
Ventilation Easy
Ventilation Difficult
Continue case with mask ventilation. MAINTAIN CRICOID PRESSURE
Administer Anesthesia Deliver Baby
Modified with permission from reference 91.

Antihypertensive Drugs Used to Prevent or Treat Hypertension during General Anesthesia

Drug	Administration and Dose	Onset and Duration of Action	Effect on Uterine and Placental Blood Flow	Special Properties: Advantages	Special Properties: Disadvantages
Hydralazine Arteriolar vasodilator	IV bolus: 5-10 mg	Maximum effect requires 20-30 min after IV administration; duration about 2 hr	Originally thought to improve, this now questioned	1. Easy to administer; no special equipment or monitoring required 2. Maintains maternal cardiac output 3. Long history of safe use in obstetrics	1. Slow unreliable onset 2. Maternal tachycardia 3. Decreased placental blood flow; fetal distress 4. Neonatal thrombocytopenia 5. Maternal nausea
Labetalol β and α blocker ?-β2 agonist	IV boluses: 10-20 mg up to total of 1-3 mg/kg	IV onset, 1-2 min; duration 2-3 hr	Improves uterine and placental blood flow	1. Easy to administer; no special equipment or monitoring 2. Little risk of overshoot 3. No associated fetal bradycardia or distress 4. Improved placental blood flow 5. Few maternal side effects 6. Rapid onset 7. Becoming widely used by obstetricians and anesthesiologists	1. Large variation in effective dose 2. Alone, may not effectively decrease BP 3. Use with caution in patients with asthma, COPD, or compromised ventricular function
Nitroglycerin Venodilator	Constant IV infusion: 5-50 µg/min Infusion: 25-50 mg/500 ml (50-100 µg/ml)	Onset less than 2 min; duration only a few minutes	Questionable, depends on state of maternal hydration; has been associated with fetal deterioration	1. Rapid onset and dissipation	1. Need IV pump to administer 2. Should make up in glass 3. May need arterial line 4. Great variation in response

Drug	Administration and Dose	Onset and Duration of Action	Effect on Uterine and Placental Blood Flow	Special Properties: Advantages	Special Properties: Disadvantages
Trimethaphan Ganglionic blocker	IV boluses: 1-4 mg IV infusion: 0.3 - 6 mg/min (1 mg/ml)	IV onset less than 1 min; duration less 5 min	Minimal, if no severe maternal hypotension	1. Reliable-rapid acting 2. Large molecular weight limits fetal transfer 3. Rapid dissipation	1. May require arterial line for BP monitoring 2. Interferes with action of pseudocholinesterase, resulting in prolonged duration of succinylcholine 3. Histamine release (?) 4. May cause mydriasis
Nitroprusside Direct-acting arterial vasodilator	Constant IV infusion: 0.15-10 μg/kg/min Infusion: 50 mg/500 ml 5% dextrose in water (100 μg/ml)	Onset less than 1 min; duration only a few minutes	Dilates uterine artery in vitro; no ill effects unless severe hypotension present	1. Rapid onset and dissipation 2. Potent reliable antihypertensive 3. No ill effects on fetus	1. Unstable solution, must protect from light 2. Easy to overshoot; need arterial line 3. Difficult to regulate 4. Increased intracranial pressure 5. Cyanide toxicity; not a problem with short-term use and infusion <3μg/kg/min 6. Tachyphylaxis

Reproduced with permission from reference 91.

Regional Anesthetic Techniques in Obstetrics for Labor and Vaginal Delivery

Technique	Example	Area of Anesthesia
Infiltration	Local for episiotomy	Perineal skin and subcutaneous tissue
	Local for cesarean section	Skin, subcutaneous tissue fascia, peritoneum
Peripheral neural blockade		
Single nerve	Pudendal	S2 - S4
Plexus	Lumbar sympathetic	T10 - L1
	Paracervical	T10 - L1
Central neural blockade		
Epidural	Lumbar	
	Standard	T10 - S5
	Segmental	T10 - L1
	Caudal	
	Standard	T10 - S5
	High catheter	T10 - S5
	Low catheter	S2 - S5
	Combined	
	Segmental	T10 - L1
	+	+
	Low caudal	S2 - S5
Subarachnoid	Standard	T10 - S5
	Low (saddle)	S1 - S5

Reproduced with permission from reference 91.

Drugs Used for Spinal and Epidural Anesthesia for Cesarean Section

Spinal

Drug	Dosage Range (mg)	Duration (min)
Lidocaine	60 - 75	45 - 75
Bupivacaine	7.5 - 15.0	60 - 120
Tetracaine	7.0 - 10.0	60 - 120
Procaine	100 - 150	30 - 60
Adjuvant Drugs		
Epinephrine	0.2	
Morphine	0.25 - 0.4	360 - 1080
Fentanyl	0.0125 - 0.025	180 - 420

Epidural

Drug	Dosage Range (mg)	Duration (min)
Lidocaine 2% with epinephrine	300 - 500	75 - 100
2-Chloroprocaine 3%	450 - 750	40 - 50
Bupivacaine 0.5%	75 - 125	120 - 180
Adjuvant Drugs		
Morphine	3 - 5	720 - 1440
Fentanyl	0.05 0.10	120 - 240
Meperidine	50 - 75	240 - 720

Modified with permission from reference 84.

Clinical Features of Epidural, Subdural, and Spinal blocks

Feature	Epidural block	Subdural block	Spinal block
Onset time	Slow	Slow	Rapid
Spread	As expected	Higher than expected; may extend intracranially, but sacral sparing is common	Higher than expected; may extend intracranially, and a sacral block is usually present
Nature of block	Segmental	Patchy	Dense
Motor block	Minimal	Minimal	Dense
Hypotension	Less than spinal and dependent on the extent of the block	Less than spinal and dependent on the extent of the block	Likely

Reproduced with permission from reference 82.

Sedatives and Nonopioid Adjuncts Used for Labor

Class	Drug	Usual dose	Onset	Duration	Comments
Barbiturates	Pentobarbital (Nembutal)	100 - 200 mg PO/IM	30 - 60 min		Possible antianalgesic effect if used alone
	Secobarbital (Seconal)	100 mg PO/IM			Useful only in very early or latent phase labor
Phenothiazines	Promethazine (Phenergan)	25 mg IV/ 50 mg IM	20 min	4 - 5 hr	Possible contribution to maternal hypotension, anti-emetic effect, wide use in combination with opioids
	Propiomazine (Largon)	20 - 40 mg IV/IM	15 - 30 min IV, 40 - 60 min IM	1 - 2 hr IV, 3 - 4 hr IM	Shorter onset and duration than promethazine, maternal hypotension, respiratory depression greater than with promethazine
Antihistamines	Hydroxyzine (Vistaril)	50 mg IM	30 min	4 hr	Use to prevent nausea and vomiting with opioids, painful on injection, no IV formulation
Benzodiazepines	Diazepam (Valium)	2 - 5 mg IV/ 10 mg IM	5 min	1 - 2 hr/3 - 4 hr	Use as treatment for eclamptic seizures, an active metabolite, prolonged half-life in neonate, neonatal depression possibly prolonged, neonatal hypotonia and impaired thermogenesis, rare use in labor
	Lorazepam (Ativan)	1 - 2 mg IV/ 2 - 4 mg IM	20 - 40 min	6 - 8 hr	Shorter elimination half-life but longer clinical effect-not used in obstetrics
	Midazolam (Versed)	1 - 5 mg IV in increments	3 - 5 min	1 - 2 hr	Water soluble, good amnesia, short half-life, not used for labor-primarily adjunct after cesarean delivery
Dissociative	Ketamine (Ketalar)	10 - 20 mg IV increments, up to 1 mg/kg over 30 minutes	30 - 60 sec	5 min	Psychomimetic effects with higher doses, not useful for first-stage labor, used just before delivery or as an adjunct to regional anesthesia, higher doses possibly leading to loss of consciousness and increased uterine tone

PO, Oral; IM, intramuscular; IV intravenous.

Reproduced with permission from reference 91.

Local Anesthetics and Opioids Commonly Used for Intermittent Bolus Injection Labor Epidural Analgesia

Concentration	Total Dose	Opioid	Result	Indications
Bupivacaine				
0.5%	5 - 10 ml	None	Profound sensory block Profound analgesia Good motor block	Painful labors "Trial of forceps" Midforceps rotation
0.25%	10 - 15 ml	None	Good sensory block Good analgesia Some motor block	Painful labors Malrotation
0.25%	5 - 10 ml	Fentanyl 1 - 3 µg/ml, Sufentanil 0.1 - 0.5 µg/ml	Profound sensory block Profound analgesia Some motor block	Painful labors "Trial of forceps" Midforceps rotation
0.125%	10 - 15 ml	Fentanyl 1 - 3 µg/ml	Good sensory block Good analgesia Some motor block	Normal labors Outlet forceps
0.03 - 0.06%	10 - 15 ml	Sufentanil 0.1 - 0.5 µg/ml	Little sensory block Good analgesia No motor block	Normal labors Outlet forceps

Lidocaine				
1 - 2%	10 - 20 ml	None (usually). may add fentanyl or sufentanil	Profound sensory block Profound analgesia Good motor block	Painful labors "Trial of forceps" Midforceps rotation Postpartum procedures
2-Chloroprocaine				
2 - 3%	10 - 20 ml	None	Profound sensory block Profound analgesia Good motor block	Fetal distress "Trial of forceps" Midforceps rotation

Reproduced with permission from reference 93.

Local Anesthetics and Opioids Commonly Used for Continuous Infusion Labor Epidural Analgesia

Concentration	Total Dose	Opioid	Result	Indications
Bupivacaine				
0.5%	5 - 10 ml/h	None	Profound sensory block Profound analgesia Good motor block	Extremely painful labors Planned instrumental delivery
0.25%	10 - 15 ml/h	None	Good sensory block Good analgesia Some motor block	Painful labors ? Instrumental delivery ? Preeclampsia
0.25%	5 - 10 ml/h	Fentanyl 1 - 3 μg/ml, Sufentanil 0.1 - 0.5 μg/ml	Profound sensory block Profound analgesia Some motor block	Painful labors ? Instrumental delivery ? Preeclampsia
0.125%	10 - 15 ml/h	Fentanyl 1 - 3 μg/ml	Good sensory block Good analgesia Some motor block	Normal labors ? Instrumental deliver
0.03 - 0.06%	10 - 15 ml/h	Sufentanil 0.1 - 0.5 μg/ml	Little sensory block Good analgesia No motor block	Normal labors Early labor

Lidocaine				
0.25 - 0.5%	7 - 15 ml/h	None (usually). may add fentanyl or sufentanil	Profound sensory block Profound analgesia Good motor block	Painful labors Planned instrumental delivery Postpartum procedures
2-Chloroprocaine				
0.5 - 1.0%	7 - 15 ml/h	None	Profound sensory block Profound analgesia Good motor block	Fetal distress "Trial of forceps" Midforceps rotation

Reproduced with permission from reference 93.

Local Anesthetics Commonly Used for Cesarean Section with Subarachnoid Block

	Lidocaine 5% in 7.5% Dextrose	Tetracaine 1% in Equal Volume of 10% Dextrose	Bupivacaine 0.75% in 8.25% Dextrose
Dosage (mg) according to height (cm):			
150 - 160	65	8	8
160 - 182	70	9	10
182 and taller	75	10	12
Onset of action (min)	1 - 3	3 - 5	2 - 4
Duration of action (min)	45 - 75	120 - 180	120 - 180

Reproduced with permission from reference 94.

Intrathecal and Epidural Opiates as Adjuvants for Intraoperative and Postoperative Pain Relief in Cesarean Section

Drug	Predelivery Dose		Postdelivery Dose		Onset (min)	Duration with Epinephrine 1:200,000 (hr)
	Subarachnoid (μg)	Epidural (μg)	Subarachnoid (μg)	Epidural (μg)		
Fentanyl	10 - 15	50 - 75	-	50 - 100	5 - 8	2 - 3
Sufentanil	5 - 10	20 - 30	-	30 - 50	5 - 8	5 - 7
Morphine	250 - 300	-	-	4000 - 5000	40 - 50	16 - 24

Reproduced with permission from reference 84.

Opioids Used for Labor Analgesia

Drug	Usual dose (IV/IM)	Onset (IV/IM)	Duration	Comments
Meperidine	25 mg IV/ 50 mg IM	5 - 10 min IV/ 40 - 45 min IM	2 - 3 hr	Active metabolite in normeperidine, neonatal effects most likely if delivery occurs between 1 and 4 hr after administration
Morphine	2 - 5 mg IV/ 10 mg IM	5 min IV/ 20 - 40 min IM	3 - 4 hr	Infrequent use during labor, greater respiratory depression in neonate than with meperidine
Fentanyl	25 - 50 μg IV/ 100 μg IM	2 - 3 min IV/ 10 min IM	30 - 60 min	Short acting, potent respiratory depressant, used as continuous infusion and/or PCA, cumulative effect with large doses over time
Nalbuphine	10 - 20 mg IV/IM	2 - 3 min IV/ 15 min IM/SQ	3 - 6 hr	Agonist/antagonist, less nausea and vomiting than with meperidine
Butorphanol	1 - 2 mg IV/IM	5 - 10 min IV/IM	3 - 4 hr	Agonist/antagonist, maternal sedation similar to meperidine plus phenothiazine
Pentazocine	20 - 40 mg IV/IM	2 - 3 min IV/ 15 - 20 min IM/SQ	2 - 3 hr	Agonist/antagonist, psychomimetic effects possible with usual doses but more frequent after large doses, infrequent use

IV, Intravenous; IM, intramuscular; PCA, patient-controlled analgesia; SQ, subcutaneous.

Reproduced with permission from reference 91.

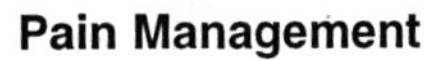

Pain Management

Organizational Aspects of an Anesthesiology-based Postoperative Pain Program

1. Education (initial, updates)
   - Anesthesiologists
   - Surgeons
   - Nurses
   - Pharmacists
   - Patients and families
   - Hospital administrators
   - Health insurance carriers
2. Areas of regular administrative activity
   - Maintenance of clear lines of communication
   - Human resources: 24-hour a day availability of pain service personnel
   - Evaluation (including safety) of equipment (e.g., pumps)
   - Secretarial support
   - Economic issues
   - Continuing quality improvement (CQI)
   - Resident physician teaching (if applicable)
   - Pain management-related research (if applicable)
3. Collaboration with nursing services
   - Job description for pain service nurse (if applicable)
   - Nursing policies and procedures
   - Nurses' in-service and continuing education
   - Definition of roles in patient care
   - Institutional administrative activities
   - Continuing quality improvement (CQI)
   - Research activities (if applicable)
4. Elements of documentation
   - Preprinted orders
   - Policies
   - Procedures
   - Bedside pain management flow sheet
   - Daily consultation notes
   - Educational packages

Reprinted with permission from reference 95.

Practice Guidelines for Acute Pain Management in the Perioperative Setting

Information Recorded on a Bedside Pain Management Flow Sheet

1. Patient assessment at regular intervals
   According to institutional protocols (e.g., pain levels, respiratory evaluation, sedation)*
2. Medication administration
   Intravenous PCA
      Incremental dose
      Lockout interval
      1 or 4 h limit
      Rate of continuous infusion (if applicable)
      Supplemental doses for breakthrough pain
      Total drug use per unit of time (e.g., nursing shift end total)
   Epidural analgesia
      Bolus dose and time (if applicable)
      Infusion rate (if applicable)
      Supplemental doses for breakthrough pain

PCA = patient-controlled analgesia.

*These and other observations may be documented on a separate Vital Signs Flow Sheet.

Reprinted with permission from reference 95.

Preprinted Daily Clinical Note Form

TECHNIQUE

PCA

Opioid: ❑ morphine ❑ meperidine ❑ hydromorphone ❑ other ______________________

Concentration: _____ mg/ml

Incremental dose _____ mg Lockout _____ min

Infusion _____ mg/h ❑ Continuous ❑ Night only

Total opioid use _____ mg/8 h

Epidural

❑ Bolus _____ mg/ _____ h ❑ Infusion _____ ml/h

Opioid

❑ Morphine (1 mg/ml) ❑ Meperidine (2 mg/ml) ❑ Fentanyl (4 µg/ml) ❑ Other _____

Local anesthetic

❑ Bupivacaine 0.0625% ❑ Bupivacaine 0.125% ❑ Other _____

Other care ____

Problem-oriented history and physical examination

Pain levels (0-10 scale)

At rest _____ With activity _____ ❑ Patient unable to report

Patient satisfied with current pain management ❑ Yes ❑ No

Epidural catheter
Site clean and nontender ❑ Yes ❑ No
❑ Removed intact

Vital signs
Satisfactory ❑ Yes ❑ No

Neurologic function
Sensory or motor block is limiting function ❑ Yes ❑ No

Side effects: (0 = absent; 1 = present, no treatment needed; 2 = present, treatment effective; 3 = present, treatment not effective)
Respiratory depression _____ N & V _____ Pruritus _____
Urinary retention _____ Sedation _____

Treatment plan
❑ Continue present therapy to maintain control of severe pain.
❑ Modify present therapy to improve control of severe pain.
❑ Discontinue present therapy; analgesia to be provided by primary care team.

Comments ____
____
____
____

Patient seen and examined.

Date _____ Time _____ Signature ______________________________ M.D.

Reprinted with permission from reference 95.

Important Elements of Intravenous PCA Preprinted Orders

1. Drug(s), concentration(s)
2. Pump settings
   - Incremental dose
   - Lockout interval
   - Other limits (e.g., 4 h, 1 h)
3. Mode of use (PCA only, Continuous infusion)
4. Initial drug loading instructions
5. Instructions for treating breakthrough pain
6. A statement to eliminate the ordering of CNS depressants by others
7. Monitoring instructions
8. Availability of drugs to treat side effects
9. Instructions for treatment of side effects
   - Respiratory depression
   - Nausea and/or vomiting
   - Pruritus
   - Urinary retention
10. Instructions about concurrent use of other CNS depressants
11. Instructions for whom to contact if problems occur
12. Date, time, signature

PCA = patient-controlled analgesia; CNS = central nervous system.

Reprinted with permission from reference 95.

Elements of Intravenous PCA Daily Care by Anesthesiologists

The following items should be included during a bedside evaluation at least once a day while iv PCA is administered.

1. Note the dose of analgesic medication given in the past 24 h, and parameters of PCA settings (PCA bolus dose, lockout interval, basal infusion [if applicable], hourly or other interval limit).
2. Evaluate pain intensity both at rest and with operation-specific convalescent activity (e.g., passive continuous movement for knee replacement or chest physical therapy for thoracotomy). If pain is out of proportion to the surgical procedure, the number of days elapsed postoperatively, and analgesic therapy given, consider whether another cause is present (e.g., surgical complication, personality disorder, opioid tolerance) and initiate appropriate evaluation, including communication with the surgeon and/or other consultant physicians.
3. Determine whether side effects are present. Assess each side effect in the context of the type of operation and days elapsed since the operation. Decide whether the side effect is in proportion to the operation, the number of days postoperatively, and the amount of opioid and other medications given. For sedation, as an example, note other concurrent drug therapy and decide whether to undertake additional workup (e.g., glucose, electrolytes, arterial blood gas, calcium, magnesium, electrocardiogram).
4. Perform a problem-oriented physical examination (e.g., surgical site, presence of rales, venous thrombosis). Note the current vital signs (HR, RR, BP) and compare them with the last evaluation. If these are unstable or unsatisfactory (e.g., low BP or irregular pulse), consider suitable diagnostic workup (e.g., hematocrit, electrocardiogram).
5. Consider whether the patient would benefit from changing the PCA pump settings or the PCA opioid.
6. Note concurrent medications and consider whether the patient would benefit from changing the overall regimen (e.g., simplifying to avert drug interactions), or employing adjuvant analgesic medication or nonpharmacologic therapies, and if so, order these.
7. Evaluate overall patient satisfaction with current care.
8. Evaluate patient's response(s) to prior adjustments of pain therapy or addition of adjuvants (e.g., for nausea or anxiety).
9. Evaluate patient's suitability for making the transition to simpler alternatives (e.g., oral analgesics).
10. Discuss the assessment and plan with the patient and the patient's nurse and/or surgeon, when appropriate.
11. Document findings, impression, and plan in the hospital chart.
12. Ensure availability of personnel with appropriate expertise to deal with questions or problems at any time.

PCA = patient-controlled analgesia; HR = heart rate; RR = respiratory rate; BP = blood pressure.

Reprinted with permission from reference 95.

Elements of Epidural Analgesia Daily Care by Anesthesiologists

The following items should be included during a bedside evaluation at least once a day while epidural analgesia is administered.

1. Note the dose of analgesic medication given in the past 24 h, and present parameters of bolus administration or infusion pump settings (if used).
2. Evaluate pain intensity both at rest and with operation-specific convalescent activity (e.g., passive continuous movement for knee replacement or chest physical therapy for thoracotomy). If pain is out of proportion to the surgical procedure, the number of days elapsed postoperatively, and analgesic therapy given, consider whether another cause is present (e.g., surgical complication, personality disorder, opioid tolerance) and initiate appropriate evaluation, including communication with the surgeon and/or consultant physicians.
3. Determine whether side effects are present. Assess each side effect in the context of the type of operation and days elapsed since the operation. Decide whether the side effect is in proportion to the operation, the number of days postoperatively, and amount of opioid and other medications given. For sedation, as an example, note other concurrent drug therapy, as well as the patient's physical status, and decide whether to undertake other workup (e.g., glucose, electrolytes, arterial blood gas, calcium, magnesium, electrocardiogram).
4. Perform a problem-oriented physical examination (e.g., surgical site, presence of rales, venous thrombosis, sensory/motor function). Included in the physical examination should be an examination of the catheter site and brief necrologic evaluation for evidence of catheter-related complications (e.g., change in position, infection, hematoma), as well as an evaluation for cardiovascular stability (especially in patients receiving local anesthetics). Note the current vital signs (HR, RR, BP) and compare them with the last evaluation. If these are unstable or unsatisfactory, consider suitable diagnostic workup (e.g., hematocrit, electrocardiogram).
5. Adjust drug doses, administration interval, infusion pump settings, or change to a different analgesic, as appropriate.
6. Note concurrent medications and consider whether the patient would benefit from changing the overall regimen (e.g., simplifying to avert drug interactions), or employing adjuvant analgesic medications or nonpharmacologic therapies, and if so, order these.
7. Evaluate overall patient satisfaction, with current care.

Elements of Epidural Analgesia Daily Care by Anesthesiologists (continued)

8. Evaluate the patient's response(s) to prior adjustments of pain therapy or addition of adjuvants (e.g., for nausea or anxiety). Make changes in pain and adjuvant therapy as indicated.
9. Evaluate the patient's suitability for making the transition to simpler alternatives (e.g., oral analgesics).
10. Discuss the assessment and plan with the patient and patient's nurse and/or surgeon, when appropriate.
11. Document findings, impression, and plan in the hospital chart.
12. Ensure availability of personnel with appropriate expertise to deal with questions or problems at any time.

HR = heart rate; RR = respiratory rate; BP = blood pressure.

Reprinted with permission from reference 95.

Important Elements of Epidural Analgesia Preprinted Orders

1. Drug(s), concentration(s)
2. Instructions for administration
   - If boluses
     - Drug dose
     - Interval between injections
   - If infusion
     - Loading dose
     - Infusion rate
3. Instructions for treating breakthrough pain
4. Maintain iv route and access to drugs for immediate use
5. A statement to eliminate the ordering of CNS depressants by others
6. Monitoring instruction
   - For effects of opioids
   - For effects of local anesthetics
     - Bradycardia
     - Hypotension
     - Extensive sensory or motor block
7. Observations that should be communicated to the anesthesiologist (e.g., systolic blood pressure less than ___ mmHg)
8. Instructions for treatment of side effects
   - Respiratory depression
   - Nausea and/or vomiting
   - Pruritus
   - Urinary retention
9. Instructions about concurrent use of other CNS depressants
10. Instructions for whom to contact if problems occur
11. Date, time, signature

CNS = central nervous system.

Reprinted with permission from reference 95.

Considerations in Making the Transition of Pain Therapy from More Sophisticated Techniques (e.g., PCA, EA, RA) to Less Sophisticated Techniques (e.g., oral analgesics)

1. Review the efficacy and dose requirement of the sophisticated technique.
2. Consider the pain expected following the transition: type of procedure, level of activity (including physical therapy), and other sources of discomfort (e.g., nasogastric tube).
3. Review the patient's past experience with oral analgesics. What has been effective? What has caused side effects?
4. Based on the above information, use the simple technique with an analgesic drug and dose calculated to provide adequate analgesia. Adjust the dose as needed based on regular assessment.
5. Overlap therapy during the transition, i.e., do not discontinue the original therapy until the replacement has reached a therapeutic effect.
6. Provide for treatment of "breakthrough" pain during use of the simpler method.
7. If there is to be a change in responsibility for prescribing an analgesic (e.g., the surgeon assumes responsibility for an oral analgesic), be sure the change is clearly understood and that orders are available from the new therapist.

PCA = patient-controlled analgesia; EA = epidural analgesia; RA = regional analgesic techniques.

Reprinted with permission from reference 95.

Opioid Analgesics Used to Manage Cancer Pain*

Generic Name	Proprietary Name	Route	Dose Equivalence†,‡ (mg)	Comments
Opioids conventionally used to manage mild to moderate pain				
Codeine	Various	Oral	200	With the exception of codeine,
Dihydrocodeine	Various	Oral		these opioids are compounded
Hydrocodone	Vicodin, Lortab, various	Oral		with aspirin or acetaminophen,
Oxycodone	Various	Oral		which imposes a dosage ceiling.
Opioids conventionally used to manage moderate to severe pain				
"Immediate release" morphine	MSIR	Oral	30	Especially useful for initial dose titration and prn supplementation with long-acting opioids
Controlled release morphine	MS Contin, Oramorph	Oral	30	Used around-the clock for basal pain (Do not break, crush, or chew.)
Morphine	Various	Parenteral	10	Usual standard for comparison
Hydromorphone	Dilaudid	Oral	7.5	Especially useful for initial dose titration and prn supplementation with long-acting opioids
Hydromorphone	Dilaudid	Parenteral	1.5	Often used subcutaneously
Oxycodone	Various	Oral	20-30	Often compounded with adjuvants for moderate pain Used as single entity for severe pain Sustained release form is available
Fentanyl	Sublimaze	Intravenous	0.1	Minimal experience outside the hospital setting

Generic Name	Proprietary Name	Route	Dose Equivalence†,‡ (mg)	Comments
Fentanyl	Duragesic	Transdermal	45-134 mg oral morphine ~25 μg/h fentanyl	Used around-the clock for stable pain, especially with GI dysfunction
Methadone	Dolophine	Oral	20	Inexpensive, but long, variable half-life may complicate titration and predispose to toxicity
Methadone	Dolophine	Parenteral	10	Inexpensive, but long, variable half-life may complicate titration and predispose to toxicity
Levorphanol	Levodromoran	Oral	4	Long half-life with much shorter dosing interval
Levorphanol	Levodromoran	Parenteral	2	Long half-life with much shorter dosing interval

*This list is partial and based on commonly used U.S. formulations. Meperidine and the agonist-antagonist opioids are not included in the table. Meperidine may produce seizures because of accumulation of the normeperidine breakdown product during chronic administration. This is of particular importance in the elderly and in patients with abnormal renal function. The agonist-antagonist opioids have ceiling and dysphoric effects and may precipitate withdrawal in patients chronically receiving pure agonist opioids.

†Dose equivalencies are approximate.

‡When converting between drugs or routes of administration, is recommended to reduce the calculated dose by 25 - 50% to account for incomplete cross-tolerance. (Based on clinical observation, methadone dose should be reduced by 75%.) Appropriate titration of dosage should then be performed as clinically indicated.

Reprinted with permission from reference 97.

Commonly Used Adjuvant Analgesics for Cancer Pain Management

Class (examples)	Usual Indications
Anticonvulsants	
Phenytoin Carbamazepine Clonazepam Valproate	Neuropathic pain, particularly lancinating or paroxysmal pain
Antidepressants	
Amitriptyline Nortriptyline Imipramine Desipramine Trazodone	Neuropathic pain
Local anesthetics	
Lidocaine Mexiletine	Neuropathic pain
Corticosteroids	
Dexamethasone Prednisone	Tumor invasion of neural tissue, elevated intracranial pressure, spinal cord compression, additional effects (mood elevation, antiemesis, appetite stimulation)
Antihistaminics	
Hydroxyzine	Coanalgesic, antiemetic
Muscle relaxants	
Orphenadrine Carisoprodol Methocarbamol Chlorzoxazone Cyclobenzaprine	Occasionally useful for musculoskeletal pain
Neuroleptics	
Methotrimeprazine Fluphenazine	Neuropathic pain
Other drugs for neuropathic pain	
Baclofen Clonidine Calcitonin Capsaicin, topical	Neuropathic pain

Class (examples)	Usual Indications
Drug action on bone	
Biphosphonates (pamidronate)	Bone pain
Calcitonin	
Radiopharmaceuticals (Strontium 89)	
Anticholinergics	
Scopolamine	Visceral pain due to bowel obstruction
Glycopyrrolate	
Psychostimulants	
Caffeine	Decrease sedation due to opioid analgesia
Methylphenidate	
Dextroamphetamine	

Reprinted with permission from reference 96.

Comparison of Antidepressants Used in Pain Management

Drug	Effect on Serotonin	Anti-cholinergic Properties	Sedative Properties	Daily Dose	Comments
Amitriptyline	+++	+	+++	15 - 200 mg	10 mg at bedtime sometimes useful if patient unable to tolerate hangover
Desipramine	0	++	+	50 - 200 mg	
Doxepin	0	+	+	10 - 150 mg	
Imipramine	++	++	++	50 - 200 mg	
Nortriptyline	+	+	++	50 - 200 mg	
Trazodone	+++	0	+++	150 - 400 mg	Priapism has been reported

0 = absent; + = mild; + + = moderate; +++ = marked.

Reprinted with permission from reference 96.

Sympathetically Maintained Pain (SMP)

That aspect of the pain which can be relieved by a local anesthetic block of the sympathetic ganglia that serve the painful area is termed sympathetically maintained pain. J N Campbell - 1996

SMP Diagnosis

Local Anesthetic Sympathetic Block

Advantages:
- "Gold Standard"
- Few false negatives with proper technique

Disadvantages:
- Invasive - special training needed
- High potential for placebo response
- Nerve palsies - Phrenic
- Pneumothorax, Cardiac arrythmias
- Vascular, epidural or intrathecal injection

Systemic α–Adrenergic Blockade with Phentolamine

Advantages:
- No somatic blockade?
- Well tolerated by patients
- Minimally invasive
- Can control for placebo effects

Disadvantages
- Variable dose
- Expense, time required
- Use with caution in cardiac disease

SMP Treatment

Pain:
- Local anesthetic sympathetic ganglion blocks
- Systemic phentolamine infusion
- Sympatholytic regional block
- Pharmacologic management
  - (neurontin, TCAs, alpha blockers?)
- Sympatholysis
  - Radiofrequency, chemical or surgical

Dysfunction:
- Aggressive physical therapy
- Psychological treatment and counseling

IASP* Definitions of Medical Terms Commonly Used to Describe Altered Sensations

Hyperalgesia
: Increased sensitivity to stimulation, excluding the special senses (includes both ailodynia and hyperalgesia)

Hypoesthesia
: Decreased sensitivity to stimulation, excluding the special senses

Hypoalgesia
: Diminished pain in response to a normally painful stimulus

Dysesthesia
: An unpleasant abnormal sensation, whether spontaneous or evoked (that is not described as painful)

Paresthesia
: An abnormal sensation, whether spontaneous or evoked

Hyperpathia
: A painful syndrome characterized by an abnormally painful reaction to a stimulus, especially a repetitive stimulus, as well as an increased threshold (the pain usually radiates and persists afler the stimulus, oflen with an abnormal delay between stimulus onset and sensation onset)

IASP = International Association for the Study of Pain

Reproduced with permisison from reference 98.

Classification: Chronic Regional Pain Syndrome (CRPS)

CRPS describes a variety of painful conditions that usually follow injury, occur regionally, have a distal predominance of abnormal findings, exceed in both magnitude and duration the expected clinical course of the inciting event, often result in significant impairment of motor function, and show variable progression over time.

CRPS Type I (RSD)

1. Follows an initiating noxious event.
2. Spontaneous pain or allodynia/hyperalgesia occurs beyond the territory of a single peripheral nerve(s), and is disproportionate to the inciting event.
3. There is or has been evidence of edema, skin blood flow abnormality, or abnormal sudomotor activity, in the region of the pain since the inciting event.
4. This diagnosis is excluded by the existence of conditions that would otherwise account for the degree of pain and dysfunction.

CRPS Type II (Causalgia)

This syndrome follows nerve injury. It is similar in all other respects to type I.

1. Is a more regionally confined presentation about a joint (e.g., ankle, knee, wrist) or area (e.g., face, eye, penis), associated with a noxious event.
2. Spontaneous pain or allodynia/hyperalgesia is usually limited to the area involved but may spread variably distal or proximal to the area, not in the territory of a dermatomal or peripheral nerve distribution.
3. Intermittent and variable edema, skin blood flow change, temperature change, abnormal sudomotor activity, and motor dysfunction, disproportionate to the inciting event, are present about the area involved.

Sympathetically Maintained Pain

Pain that is maintained by sympathetic efferent activity or neurochemical or circulating catecholamine action, as determined by pharmacological or sympathetic nerve blockade. SMP may be a feature of several types of pain disorder, and is not an essential component of any one condition. Conditions without any response to sympathetic block are, by contrast, designated as having sympathetic independent pain states (SIP).

Reproduced with permisison from reference 99.

Criteria for Differential Diagnosis of Complex Regional Pain Syndromes (CRPS) type I and II

	CRPS I	CRPS II
Etiology	Any kind of lesion	Partial nerve lesion
Localization	Distal part of extremity	Any peripheral site of body
	Independent from site of lesion	Mostly confined to the territory of affected nerve
Spreading of symptoms	Obligatory	Rare
Spontaneous pain	Common Mostly deep and superficial Orthostatic component	Obligatory Predominately superficial No orthostatic component
Mechanical allodynia	Most of patients with spreading tendency	Obligatory in nerve territory
Autonomic symptoms	Distally generalized with spreading tendency	Related to nerve lesion
Motor symptoms	Distally generalized	Related to nerve lesion
Sensory symptoms	Distally generalized with spreading tendency	Related to nerve lesion

Reproduced with permisison from reference 100.

Contrasts in Pediatric and Adult RSD

	Children	Adults
Site	Marked lower extremity predominance (5.3:1)	Upper extremity commonly involved
Spontaneous pain	Common	Common
Mechanical allodynia	Most patients	Most patients
Sex ratio	Marked female predominance (4:1)	Studies mixed
Psychological aspects	Psychiatric pathology not well documented. Possible increased tendency to RSD with psychosocial stressors	Psychiatric pathology not well documented.
Three-phase bone scan	Mixed results: use to rule out other pathology	Increased uptake of radionucleotide in the affected extremity
Treatment strategy	Resolution often possible with PT, TENS, and CBPMT	Early sympathetic block strongly advocated (Bonica 1990)
Timing of treatment	Duration of disease of little consequence in success of treatment	Early sympathetic block strongly advocated (Bonica 1990)
Technique for sympathetic block	Place catheter, run continuous infusion as inpatient	Multiple outpatient "single shot" blocks

RSD = reflex sympathetic dystrophy (CRPS Type I); PT = physical therapy; TENS = transcutaneous electrical nerve stimulation; CBPMT = cognitive and behavioral pain management techniques.

Reproduced with permisison from reference 101.

Algorithm for Diagnosis of CRPS

Pain

The diagnosis of CRPS cannot be made in the absence of pain; it is a pain syndrome. However, the characteristics of the pain may vary with the initiating event and other factors. The pain is often described as burning, and might be spontaneous or evoked in the context of hyperalgesia or allodynia. Both spontaneous and evoked pain may occur together.

History

Develops after an initiating noxious event or immobilization
Unilateral extremity onset (rarely may spread to another extremity)
Symptom onset usually within a month
Exclusion criteria
Identifiable major nerve lesion (CRPS II)
Existence of anatomic, physiologic, or psychological conditions that would otherwise account for the degree of pain and dysfunction

Symptoms (Patient Report)

A. Pain (spontaneous or evoked)
   Burning
   Aching, throbbing
B. Hyperalgesia or allodynia (at some time in the disease course) to mechanical stimuli (light touch or deep pressure), to thermal stimulation, or to joint motion
C. Associated symptoms (minor)
   Swelling
   Temperature or color: asymmetry and instability
   Sweating: asymmetry and instability
   Trophic changes: hair, nails, skin

Signs (Observed)

Hyperalgesia or allodynia (light touch, deep pressure, joint movement, cold)
Edema (if unilateral and other causes excluded)
Vasomotor changes: color, temperature instability, asymmetry
Sudomotor changes
Trophic changes in skin, joint, nail, hair
Impaired motor function (may include components of dystonia and tremor)

Criteria Required for Diagnosis of CRPS I

History of pain
plus allodynia, hyperalgesia, or hyperesthesia
plus two other signs from the above list
Characteristics of spontaneous pain
Sympathetically maintained pain (SMP)
Sympathetically independent pain (SIP)
Combined SMP + SIP

Criteria for Diagnosis of Sympathetic Dysfunction

Noninvasive tests

Surface temperature asymmetry by ≥1° C, either spontaneous or in response to provocative testing

Resting or evoked sudomotor asymmetry

Invasive tests

Sympathetic ganglion block (if equivocal, up to three may be required); will usually be considered adequate only if there is demonstrated inhibition of sympathetic mediated vasoconstriction of the involved extremity.

Systemic alpha adrenergic antagonists, placebo controlled

Neuraxial blockade above the lesion may provide useful information.

Tests of unknown pathophysiologic significance

Three-phase bone scan

Radiographic patchy demineralization

Tourniquet ischemia test

Measurements of cutaneous blood flow with laser Doppler, percutaneous oxygen partial pressure differences, and computer-assisted sensory examination are interesting but evolving technologies that require further study.

Somatosensory-evoked potential measurement is not of demonstrated utility.

Regional sympathetic blockade is not recommended for diagnostic use due to multiple physiologic actions that confound interpretation.

Reproduced with permisison from reference 102.

Tests for Efficacy of Sympathetic Block

Sympathetic Function

Skin Plethysmography and "Ice Response"

Skin Conductance Response (SCR)

Previously referred to as sympathogalvanic response (SGR), this is a simple measure of activity in sudomotor neurons. It is dependent on changes in skin conductance but is also subject to habituation.

Skin Potential Response (SPR) (PASP)

SRP reflects activity in sudomotor neurons and changes in sodium flux of the sweat glands. Measurement requires a modified ECG, and has the advantage that no external signal source is required.

The Cobalt Blue Test

Filter papers soaked in cobalt blue are applied to corresponding areas of the upper extremity. A color range from blue to pink indicates sweating.

Cold Pressor Test

In conjunction with telethermography, this test enables the sympathetic response to be monitored after a nonaffected extremity is placed in ice-cold water. The cutaneous response demonstrated by surface cooling, which under normal physiologic conditions should be followed by rewarming of the skin after 20-25 minutes, will be delayed for 45 minutes or longer in cases of dysautonomia.

Blood Flow Measurements

Occlusion Skin Plethysmography

Temperature Measurement

Contact thermistors or noncontact, passive infrared measurement on corresponding areas (fingertips) of the ipsilateral and contralateral extremities on at least three sites should register ≥34°C with adequate sympatholysis. Complete sympatholysis under normal physiological circumstances should achieve a temperature measurement at the fingertips of ≥35°C. Noncontact telethermography has the advantage of allowing regional temperature differences of 0.1°C to be measured over the total area.

Laser Doppler Flowmetry (Fluxmetry)

This technique offers an excellent, noninvasive measurement of changes in skin blood flow.

Reproduced with permisison from reference 103.

Miscellaneous

Malignant Hyperthermia

Possible Signs of Malignant Hyperthermia

Tachycardia
Muscle stiffness
Hypercarbia
Tachypnea
Respiratory and metabolic acidosis
Myoglobinuria
Cardiac arrhythmias
Fever
Unstable / rising blood pressure
Cyanosis / mottling

Diagnosis of Malignant Hyperthermia

The **most sensitive indicator** of potential MH in the OR is an unanticipated increase (e.g. doubling or tripling) of end-tidal CO_2. The increase in CO_2 may occur over a brief period of time or may develop over 10 to 20 minutes. If cardiac arrest occurs, hyperkalemia should be considered immediately.

The **most specific sign** of MH is total body rigidity.

Unexpected tachycardia, tachypnea and jaw muscle rigidity are other common signs of MH.

Respiratory and metabolic acidosis usually occur **early** in MH.

Temperature elevation is often a **late sign** of MH. Temperature change during MH is best detected by core temperature measurement (tympanic, naso or oropharyngeal, esophageal, rectal, axillary or pulmonary artery). It is suggested that core temperature be measured whenever general anesthesia is administered for other than very brief procedures.

Drugs and MH

All volatile inhalation anesthetics (including desflurane and sevoflurane) and succinylcholine are MH triggers.

Nitrous oxide, barbiturates, narcotics, tranquilizers, and amide and ester local anesthetics are safe for MH patients.

Calcium channel blockers should not be administered when dantrolene has been given.

Ketamine, propofol, etomidate, vecuronium, pancuronium and atracurium have been determined to be safe drugs for MH patients.

The new muscle relaxants mivacurium, rocuronium, pipecuronium and doxacurium are also considered safe agents. Catecholamines are safe agents.

Management and Pretreatment of MH-Susceptible (MHS) Patients

A treatment plan for MH should be available.

All facilities where general anesthesia is administered (including ambulatory surgery centers) should stock 36 vials of dantrolene sodium.

Do not use MH-triggering agents with MHS patients or their relatives.

Prophylactic dantrolene should be used with caution in patients with muscle weakness or muscle disease, as muscle weakness may be exacerbated.

Dantrolene prophylaxis may be omitted if the patient will receive sedation or regional anesthesia or general anesthesia with appropriate intra-operative monitoring (including continuous temperature and continuous end-tidal CO_2 monitoring) and dantrolene is readily available for administration.

The anesthesia machine should be prepared by changing soda lime and breathing circuit, removing or inactivating vaporizers, and flushing with oxygen or air at 10 liters/min for 10 - 20 minutes.

The MHS patient undergoing outpatient surgery may be discharged on the day of surgery if the anesthetic has been uneventful and no dantrolene has been given. A minimum of 4 hours in the PACU is suggested.

Suggested Therapy for Malignant Hyperthermia Emergency

CAUTION: This protocol may not apply to every patient and must of necessity be altered according to specific patient needs. Names of on-call physicians available to consult in MH emergencies may be obtained 24 hours a day through Malignant Hyperthermia Hotline (800) MH-HYPER (800-644-9737). Outside the United States: 1-315-428-7924.

MHAUS provides educational and technical information to patients and health care providers. All MHAUS literature is available 24-hours a day, 7 days a week through the MHAUS Fax-On-Demand system at 1-800-440-9990. For non-emergency or patient referral calls: MHAUS (203) 655-3007.

1. Immediately discontinue all inhalation anesthetics and succinylcholine. Hyperventilate with 100% oxygen at high gas flows (10 L/min or greater).

2. In the absence of blood gas analysis, bicarbonate 1 - 2 mEq/kg should be administered.

3. Dantrolene sodium should be obtained, mixed with *sterile distilled water*, and 2.5 mg/kg administered intravenously. At present, dantrolene is packaged as lyophilized preparation that contains 20 mg of dantrolene and 3 grams mannitol per vial.

4. Simultaneously, cooling should be started by all routes: surface, nasogastric lavage, intravenous cold solutions, wound, and rectally.

5. Arrhythmias will usually respond to treatment of acidosis and hyperkalemia. If they persist or are life threatening, standard anti-arrhythmic agents may be used with the exception of calcium channel blockers.

6. Administer further doses of dantrolene as necessary titrated to the heart rate, muscle rigidity and temperature. Response to dantrolene should begin to occur in minutes; if not, more drug should be administered. Although the average successful dose of dantrolene is about 2.5 mg/kg, much higher doses may be needed (10 mg/kg and more). Fortunately dantrolene does not produce significant myocardial depression at these doses.

7. Change anesthetic tubing.

8. Determine and closely monitor urine output, serum potassium, calcium, arterial blood gases, end tidal CO2, and clotting studies. Hyperkalemia is common in the acute phase of MH and should be treated with intravenous glucose and insulin.

9. Observe the patient in an ICU setting for at least 24 hours since recrudescence of MH may occur, particularly following a case that was difficult to treat.

10. Follow CK, calcium, potassium and clotting studies until such time as they return to normal (e.g., q 6 hours). Observe for DIC.

11. ECG should be obtained and followed postoperatively.

12. Monitor body temperature closely since over vigorous treatment of MH may lead to hypothermia. Temperature instability may persist for several days after the acute episode. Body temperatures of 41 to 42°C are compatible with survival and normal brain function if treated promptly.

13. Insure urine output of greater than 1 m/kg/hour. Consider CVP monitoring because of fluid shifts that may occur.

14. When the patient's condition has stabilized, convert from intravenous to oral dantrolene. Although data are not available regarding optimal doses and duration of treatment with dantrolene after an episode, the patient should probably receive a total dose of 4 mg/kg/day in divided doses for 48 hours postoperatively.

15. Counsel the patient and family regarding MH and further precautions. Refer patient to MHAUS.

Reproduced with permission from reference 104.

Miscellaneous

STANDARDS OF THE AMERICAN SOCIETY OF ANESTHESIOLOGISTS

STANDARDS OF THE AMERICAN SOCIETY OF ANESTHESIOLOGISTS

As defined in the Policy Statement on Practice Parameters, Standards are rules; e.g. minimum requirements for sound practice. They are generally accepted principles for patient management.

BASIC STANDARDS FOR PREANESTHESIA CARE

(Approved by House of Delegates on October 14, 1987)

These standards apply to all patients who receive anesthesia or monitored anesthesia care. Under unusual circumstances, e.g. extreme emergencies, these standards may be modified. When this is the case, the circumstances shall be documented in the patient's record.

Standard 1: An anesthesiologist shall be responsible for determining the medical status of the patient, developing a plan of anesthesia care, and acquainting the patient or the responsible adult with the proposed plan.

The development of an appropriate plan of anesthesia care is based upon:

1. Reviewing the medical record.
2. Interviewing and examining the patient to:
   a. Discuss the medical history, previous anesthetic experiences and drug therapy.
   b. Assess those aspects of the physical condition that might affect decisions regarding perioperative risk and management.
3. Obtaining and/or reviewing tests and consultations necessary to the conduct of anesthesia.
4. Determining the appropriate prescription of preoperative medications as necessary to the conduct of anesthesia.

The responsible anesthesiologist shall verify that the above has been properly performed and documented in the patient's record.

STANDARDS FOR BASIC ANESTHETIC MONITORING

(Approved by House of Delegates on October 21, 1986 and last amended on October 13, 1993)

These standards apply to all anesthesia care although, in emergency circumstances, appropriate life support measures take precedence. These standards may be exceeded at any time based on the judgement of the responsible anesthesiologist. They are intended to encourage quality patient care, but observing them cannot guarantee any specific patient outcome. They are subject to revision from time to time, as warranted by the evolution of technology and practice. They apply to all general anesthetics, regional anesthetics and monitored anesthesia care. This set of standards addresses only the issue of basic anesthetic monitoring, which is one component of anesthesia care. In certain rare or unusual circumstances, 1) some of these methods of monitoring may be clinically impractical, and 2) appropriate use of the described monitoring methods may fail to detect untoward clinical developments. Brief interruptions of continual monitoring† may be unavoidable. *Under extenuating circumstances, the responsible anesthesiologist may waive the requirements marked with an asterisk (*); it is recommended that when this is done, it should be so stated (including the reasons) in a note in the patient's medical record.* These standards are not intended for application to the care of the obstetrical patient in labor or in the conduct of pain management.

†Note that "continual" is defined as "repeated regularly and frequently in steady rapid succession" whereas "continuous" means "prolonged without any interruption at any time."

STANDARD I

Qualified anesthesia personnel shall be present in the room throughout the conduct of all general anesthetics, regional anesthetics and monitored anesthesia care.

OBJECTIVE
Because of the rapid changes in patient status during anesthesia, qualified anesthesia personnel shall be continuously present to monitor the patient and provide anesthesia care. In the event there is a direct known hazard, e.g., radiation, to the anesthesia personnel which might require intermittent remote observation of the patient, some provision for monitoring the patient must be made. In the event that an emergency requires the temporary absence of the person primarily responsible for the anesthetic, the best judgement of the anesthesiologist will be exercised in comparing the emergency with the anesthetized patient's condition and in the selection of the person left responsible for the anesthetic during the temporary absence.

STANDARD II

During all anesthetics, the patient's oxygenation, ventilation, circulation and temperature shall be continually evaluated.

OXYGENATION

OBJECTIVE

To ensure adequate oxygen concentration in the inspired gas and the blood during all anesthetics.

METHODS

1) Inspired gas: During every administration of general anesthesia using an anesthesia machine, the concentration of oxygen in the patient breathing system shall be measured by an oxygen analyzer with a low oxygen concentration limit alarm in use.*

2) Blood oxygenation: During all anesthetics, a quantitative method of assessing oxygenation such as pulse oximetry shall be employed.* Adequate illumination and exposure of the patient are necessary to assess color.*

VENTILATION

OBJECTIVE

To ensure adequate ventilation of the patient during all anesthetics.

METHODS

1) Every patient receiving general anesthesia shall have the adequacy of ventilation continually evaluated. While qualitative clinical signs such as chest excursion, observation of the reservoir breathing bag and auscultation of breath sounds may be useful, quantitative monitoring of the carbon dioxide content and/or volume of expired gas is strongly encouraged.

2) When an endotracheal tube is inserted its presence in the trachea must be verified by clinical assessment and by identification of carbon dioxide in the expired gas. Continual end-tidal carbon dioxide analysis, in use from the time of endotracheal tube placement, until extubation or initiating transfer to a postoperative care location, shall be performed using a quantitative method such as capnography, capnometry or mass spectroscopy.*

3) When ventilation is controlled by a mechanical ventilator, there shall be in continuous use a device that is capable of detecting disconnection of components of the breathing system. The device must give an audible signal when its alarm threshold is exceeded.

4) During regional anesthesia and monitored anesthesia care, the adequacy of ventilation shall be evaluated, at least, by continual observation of qualitative clinical signs.

CIRCULATION

OBJECTIVE

To ensure the adequacy of the patient's circulatory function during all anesthetics.

METHODS

1) Every patient receiving anesthesia shall have the electrocardiogram continuously displayed from the beginning of anesthesia until preparing to leave the anesthetizing location.*

2) Every patient receiving anesthesia shall have arterial blood pressure and heart rate determined and evaluated at least every five minutes.*

3) Every patient receiving general anesthesia shall have, in addition to the above, circulatory function continually evaluated by at least one of the following: palpation of a pulse, auscultation of heart sounds, monitoring of a tracing of intra-arterial pressure, ultrasound peripheral pulse monitoring, or pulse plethysmography or oximetry.

BODY TEMPERATURE

OBJECTIVE

To aid in the maintenance of appropriate body temperature during all anesthetics.

METHODS

There shall be readily available a means to continuously measure the patient's temperature. When changes in body temperature are intended, anticipated or suspected, the temperature shall be measured.

STANDARDS FOR POSTANESTHESIA CARE

(Approved by House of Delegates on October 12, 1988 and last amended on October 21, 1992)

These Standards apply to postanesthesia care in all locations. These Standards may be exceeded based on the judgment of the responsible anesthesiologist. They are intended to encourage quality patent care, but cannot guarantee any specific patient outcome. They are subject to revision from time to time as warranted by the evolution of technology and practice. *Under extenuating circumstances, the responsible anesthesiologist may waive the requirements marked with an asterisk (*); it is recommended that when this is done, it should be so stated (including the reasons) in a note in the patient's medical record.*

STANDARD I

ALL PATIENTS WHO HAVE RECEIVED GENERAL ANESTHESIA, REGIONAL ANESTHESIA, OR MONITORED ANESTHESIA CARE SHALL RECEIVE APPROPRIATE POSTANESTHESIA MANAGEMENT.

1. A Postanesthesia Care Unit (PACU) or an area which provides equivalent postanesthesia care shall be available to receive patients after surgery and anesthesia. All patients who receive anesthesia shall be admitted to the PACU except by specific order of the anesthesiologist responsible for the patient's care.

2. The medical aspects of care in the PACU shall be governed by policies and procedures which have been reviewed and approved by the Department of Anesthesiology.

3. The design, equipment and staffing of the PACU shall meet requirements of the facility's accrediting and licensing bodies.

STANDARD II

A PATIENT TRANSPORTED TO THE PACU SHALL BE ACCOMPANIED BY A MEMBER OF THE ANESTHESIA CARE TEAM WHO IS KNOWLEDGEABLE ABOUT THE PATIENT'S CONDITION. THE PATIENT SHALL BE CONTINUALLY EVALUATED AND TREATED DURING TRANSPORT WITH MONITORING AND SUPPORT APPROPRIATE TO THE PATIENT'S CONDITION.

STANDARD III

UPON ARRIVAL IN THE PACU, THE PATIENT SHALL BE RE-EVALUATED AND A VERBAL REPORT PROVIDED TO THE RESPONSIBLE PACU NURSE BY THE MEMBER OF THE ANESTHESIA CARE TEAM WHO ACCOMPANIES THE PATIENT.

1. The patient's status on arrival in the PACU shall be documented.

2. Information concerning the preoperative condition and the surgical/anesthetic course shall be transmitted to the PACU nurse.

3. The member of the Anesthesia Care Team shall remain in the PACU until the PACU nurse accepts responsibility for the nursing care of the patient.

STANDARD IV

THE PATIENT'S CONDITION SHALL BE EVALUATED CONTINUALLY IN THE PACU.

1. The patient shall be observed and monitored by methods appropriate to the patient's medical condition. Particular attention should be given to monitoring oxygenation, ventilation, circulation and temperature. During recovery from all anesthetics, a quantitative method of assessing oxygenation such as pulse oximetry shall be employed in the initial phase of recovery.* This is not intended for application during the recovery of the obstetrical patient in whom regional anesthesia was used for labor and vaginal delivery.

STANDARD V

A PHYSICIAN IS RESPONSIBLE FOR THE DISCHARGE OF A PATIENT FROM THE POSTANESTHESIA CARE UNIT.

1. When discharge criteria are used, they must be approved by the Department of Anesthesiology and the medical staff. They may vary depending upon whether the patient is discharged to a hospital room, to the Intensive Care unit, to a short stay unit or home.

2. In the absence of the physician responsible for the discharge, the PACU nurse shall determine that the patient meets the discharge criteria. The name of the physician accepting responsibility for discharge shall be noted on the record.

1 Refer to Standards of Post Anesthesia Nursing Practice 1992 published by ASPAN, for issues of nursing care.

ETHICAL GUIDELINES FOR THE ANESTHESIA CARE OF PATIENTS WITH DO NOT RESUSCITATE ORDERS OR OTHER DIRECTIVES THAT LIMIT TREATMENT

(Approved by House of Delegates on October 13, 1993)

These guidelines apply to competent patients and also to incompetent patients who have previously expressed their preferences.

I. Given the diversity of published opinions and cultures within our society, an essential element of preoperative preparation and perioperative care for patients with Do Not Resuscitate (DNR) orders or other directives that limit treatment is communication among involved parties. it is necessary to document relevant aspects of this communication.

II. Policies automatically suspending DNR orders or other directives that limit treatment prior to procedures involving anesthetic care may not sufficiently address a patient's rights to self-determination in a responsible and ethical manner. Such policies, if they exist, should be reviewed and revised, as necessary, to reflect the content of these guidelines.

III. Prior to procedures requiring anesthetic care, any changes in existing directives that limit treatment should be documented in the medical record. These include absolute injunctions as desired by the patient (or the patient's legal representative). When appropriate, the items that should be considered are:

A. Blood product transfusion
B. Tracheal intubation or instrumentation
C. Chest compressions and direct cardiac massage
D. Defibrillation
E. Cardiac pacing, internal or external
F. Invasive monitoring
G. Postoperative ventilatory support
H. Vasoactive drug administration

IV. When relevant, the anesthesiologist should describe and discuss the appropriate use of therapeutic modalities to correct deviations of hemodynamic and respiratory variables predictably resulting from anesthetic agents and techniques.

V. Additional issues that may be relevant to discuss are perioperative placement of naso/orogastric tubes or urinary catheters, administration of antibiotics, establishment of intravenous access, maintenance of intravascular volume with nonblood products, and treatment with supplemental oxygen.

VI. It is important to discuss and document whether there are to be any exceptions to the injunction(s) against intervention should there occur a specific recognized complication of the surgery or anesthesia.

VII. Concurrence on these issues by the primary physician (if not the surgeon of record), the surgeon and the anesthesiologist is desirable. If possible, these physicians should meet together with the patient (or the patient's legal representative) when these issues are discussed. This duty of the patient's physicians is deemed to be of such importance that it should not be delegated. Other members of the health care team who are (or will be) directly involved with the patient's care during the planned procedure should, if feasible, be included in this process.

VIII. Should conflicts arise, the following resolution processes are recommended:

A. When an anesthesiologist finds the patient's or surgeon's limitations of intervention decisions to be irreconcilable with one's own moral views, then the anesthesiologist should withdraw in a nonjudgmental fashion, providing an alternative for care in a timely fashion.

B. When an anesthesiologist finds the patient's or surgeon's limitation of intervention decisions to be a conflict with generally accepted standards of care, ethical practice or institutional policies, then the anesthesiologist should voice such concerns and present the situation to the appropriate institutional body.

C. If these alternatives are not feasible within the time frame necessary to prevent further morbidity or suffering, then in accordance with the American Medical Association's Principles of Medical Ethics, care should proceed with reasonable adherence to the patient's directive, being mindful of the patient's goals and values.

IX. A representative from the hospital's anesthesiology service should establish a liaison with surgeon and nursing services for presentation, discussion and procedural application of these guidelines. Hospital staff should be made aware of the proceedings of these discussions and the motivations for them.

X. Modification of these guidelines may be appropriate when they conflict with local standards or policies, and in those emergency situations involving incompetent patients whose intentions have not been previously expressed.

GUIDELINES FOR NONOPERATING ROOM ANESTHETIZING LOCATIONS

(Approved by House of Delegates on October 19, 1994)

These guidelines apply to all anesthesia care involving anesthesiology personnel for procedures intended to be performed in locations outside an operating room. These are minimal guidelines which may be exceeded at any time based on the judgment of the involved anesthesia personnel. These guidelines encourage quality patient care but observing them cannot guarantee any specific patient outcome. These guidelines are subject to revision from time to time, as warranted by the evolution of technology and practice.

1. There should be in each location a reliable source of oxygen adequate for the length of the procedure. There should also be a backup supply. Prior to administering any anesthetic, the anesthesiologist should consider the capabilities, limitations and accessibility of both the primary and backup oxygen sources. Oxygen piped from a central source, meeting applicable codes, is strongly encouraged. The backup system should include the equivalent of at least a full E cylinder.

2. There should be in each location an adequate and reliable source of suction. Suction apparatus that meets operating room standards is strongly encouraged.

3. In any location in which inhalation anesthetics are administered, there should be an adequate and reliable system for scavenging waste anesthetic gases.

4. There should be in each location: (a) a self-inflating hand resuscitator bag capable of administering at least 90 percent oxygen as a means to deliver positive pressure ventilation; (b) adequate anesthesia drugs, supplies and equipment for the intended anesthesia care; and (c) adequate monitoring equipment to allow adherence to the "Standards for Basic Anesthetic Monitoring." In any location in which inhalation anesthesia is to be administered, there should be an anesthesia machine equivalent in function to that employed in operating rooms and maintained to current operating room standards.

5. There should be in each location, sufficient electrical outlets to satisfy anesthesia machine and monitoring equipment requirements, including clearly labeled outlets connected to an emergency power supply. In any anesthetizing location determined by the health care facility to be a "wet location" (e.g. for cytoscopy or arthroscopy or a birthing room in labor and delivery), either isolated electric power or electric circuits with ground fault circuit interrupters should be provided.*

6. There should be in each location, provision for adequate illumination of the patient, anesthesia machine (when present) and monitoring equipment. In addition, a form of battery-powered illumination other than a laryngoscope should be immediately available.

7. There should be in each location, sufficient space to accommodate necessary equipment and personnel and to allow expeditious access to the patient, anesthesia machine (when present) and monitoring equipment.

8. There should be immediately available in each location, an emergency cart with defibrillator, emergency drugs and other equipment adequate to provide cardiopulmonary resuscitation.

9. There should be immediately available in each location, a reliable means of two-way communication to request assistance.

10. For each location, all applicable building and safety codes and facility standards, where they exist, should be observed.

*See National Fire Protection Association, Health Care Facilities Code 99, Quincy, MA: NFPA, 1993.

GUIDELINES FOR REGIONAL ANESTHESIA IN OBSTETRICS

(Approved by House of Delegates on October 12, 1988 and last amended on October 30, 1991)

These guidelines apply to the use of regional anesthesia or analgesia in which local anesthetics are administered to the parturient during labor and delivery. They are intended to encourage quality patient care but cannot guarantee any specific patient outcome. Because the availability of anesthesia resources may vary, members are able for interpreting and establishing the guidelines for their own institutions response and practices. These guidelines are subject to revision from time to time as warranted by the evolution of technology and practice.

GUIDELINE I

REGIONAL ANESTHESIA SHOULD BE INITIATED AND MAINTAINED ONLY IN LOCATIONS IN WHICH APPROPRIATE RESUSCITATION EQUIPMENT AND DRUGS ARE IMMEDIATELY AVAILABLE TO MANAGE PROCEDURALLY RELATED PROBLEMS.

Resuscitation equipment should include, but is not limited to: sources of oxygen and suction, equipment to maintain an airway and perform endotracheal intubation, a means to provide positive pressure ventilation, and drugs and equipment for cardiopulmonary resuscitation.

GUIDELINE II

REGIONAL ANESTHESIA SHOULD BE INITIATED BY A PHYSICIAN WITH APPROPRIATE PRIVILEGES AND MAINTAINED BY OR UNDER THE MEDICAL DIRECTION[1] OF SUCH AN INDIVIDUAL.

Physicians should be approved through the institutional credentialing process to initiate and direct the maintenance of obstetric anesthesia and to manage procedurally related complications.

GUIDELINE III

REGIONAL ANESTHESIA SHOULD NOT BE ADMINISTERED UNTIL: (1) THE PATIENT HAS BEEN EXAMINED BY A QUALIFIED INDIVIDUAL[2]; AND (2) THE MATERNAL AND FETAL STATUS AND PROGRESS OF LABOR HAVE BEEN EVALUATED BY A PHYSICIAN WITH PRIVILEGES IN OBSTETRICS WHO IS READILY AVAILABLE TO SUPERVISE THE LABOR AND MANAGE ANY OBSTETRIC COMPLICATIONS THAT MAY ARISE.

Under circumstances defined by department protocol, qualified personnel may perform the initial pelvic examination. The physician responsible for the patient's obstetrical care should be informed of her status so that a decision can be made regarding present risk and further management.[2]

GUIDELINE IV

AN INTRAVENOUS INFUSION SHOULD BE ESTABLISHED BEFORE THE INITIATION OF REGIONAL ANESTHESIA AND MAINTAINED THROUGHOUT THE DURATION OF THE REGIONAL ANESTHETIC.

GUIDELINE V

REGIONAL ANESTHESIA FOR LABOR AND/OR VAGINAL DELIVERY REQUIRES THAT THE PARTURIENT'S VITAL SIGNS AND THE FETAL HEART RATE BE MONITORED AND DOCUMENTED BY A QUALIFIED INDIVIDUAL. ADDITIONAL MONITORING APPROPRIATE TO THE CLINICAL CONDITION OF THE PARTURIENT AND THE FETUS SHOULD BE EMPLOYED WHEN INDICATED. WHEN EXTENSIVE REGIONAL BLOCKADE IS ADMINISTERED FOR COMPLICATED VAGINAL DELIVERY, THE STANDARDS FOR BASIC ANESTHETIC MONITORING[3] SHOULD BE APPLIED.

GUIDELINES VI

REGIONAL ANESTHESIA FOR CESAREAN DELIVERY REQUIRES THAT THE STANDARDS FOR BASIC ANESTHETIC MONITORING BE APPLIED AND THAT A PHYSICIAN WITH PRIVILEGES IN OBSTETRICS BE IMMEDIATELY AVAILABLE.

GUIDELINES VII

QUALIFIED PERSONNEL, OTHER THAN THE ANESTHESIOLOGIST ATTENDING THE MOTHER, SHOULD BE IMMEDIATELY AVAILABLE TO ASSUME RESPONSIBILITY FOR RESUSCITATION OF THE NEWBORN.[3]

The primary responsibility of the anesthesiologist is to provide care to the mother. If the anesthesiologist is also requested to provide brief assistance in the care of the newborn, the benefit to the child must be compared to the risk to the mother.

GUIDELINES VIII

A PHYSICIAN WITH APPROPRIATE PRIVILEGES SHOULD REMAIN READILY AVAILABLE DURING THE REGIONAL ANESTHETIC TO MANAGE ANESTHETIC COMPLICATIONS UNTIL THE PATIENT'S POSTANESTHESIA CONDITION IS SATISFACTORY AND STABLE.

GUIDELINE IX

ALL PATIENTS RECOVERING FROM REGIONAL ANESTHESIA SHOULD RECEIVE APPROPRIATE POSTANESTHESIA CARE. FOLLOWING CESAREAN DELIVERY AND/OR EXTENSIVE REGIONAL BLOCKADE, THE STANDARDS FOR POSTANESTHESIA CARE[4] SHOULD BE APPLIED.

1. A postanesthesia care unit (PACU) should be available to receive patients. The design, equipment and staffing should meet requirements of the facility's accrediting and licensing bodies.

2. When a site other than the PACU is used, equivalent postanesthesia care should be provided.

GUIDELINES X

THERE SHOULD BE A POLICY TO ASSURE THE AVAILABILITY IN THE FACILITY OF A PHYSICIAN TO MANAGE COMPLICATIONS AND TO PROVIDE CARDIOPULMONARY RESUSCITATION FOR PATIENTS RECEIVING POSTANESTHESIA CARE.

1 The Anesthesia Care Team (Approved by ASA House of Delegates 10/26/82 and last amended 10/25/95).

2 Guidelines for Perinatal Care (American Academy of Pediatrics and American College of Obstetricians and Gynecologists, 1988.)

3 Standards for Basic Anesthetic Monitoring (Approved by ASA House of Delegates 10/21/86 and last amended 10/25/95).

4 Standards for Postanesthesia Care (Approved by ASA House of Delegates 10/12/88 and last amended 10/19/94).

GUIDELINES FOR PATIENT CARE IN ANESTHESIOLOGY

(Approved by House of Delegates on October 3, 1967 and last amended on October 16, 1985)

I. Definition of Anesthesiology:
Anesthesiology is a discipline within the practice of medicine specializing in:

A. The medical management of patients who are rendered unconscious and/or insensible to pain and emotional stress during surgical, obstetrical and certain other medical procedures (involves preoperative, intraoperative and postoperative evaluation and treatment of these patients);

B. The protection of life functions and vital organs (e.g., brain, heart, lungs, kidneys, liver) under the stress of anesthetic, surgical and other medical procedures;

C. The management of problems in pain relief.

D. The management of cardiopulmonary resuscitation;

E. The management of problems in pulmonary care;

F. The management of critically ill patients in special care unit.

II. Anesthesiologist's Responsibilities:

Anesthesiologists are physicians who, after college, have graduated from an accredited medical school and have successfully completed an approved residency in anesthesiology. Anesthesiologists' responsibilities to patients should include:

A. Preanesthetic evaluation and treatment;

B. Medical management of patients and their anesthetic procedures;

C. Postanesthetic evaluation and treatment:

D. On-site medical direction of any nonphysician who assists in the technical aspects of anesthesia care to the patient.

III. Guidelines for Anesthesia Care:

A. The same quality of anesthetic care should be available for all patients:
1. 24 hours a day, seven days a week;
2. Emergency as well as elective patients;
3. Obstetrical, medical and surgical patients.

B. Preanesthetic evaluation and preparation means that the responsible anesthesiologist:
   1. Reviews the chart.
   2. Interviews the patient to:
      a. Discuss medical history, including anesthetic experiences and drug therapy.
      b. Perform any examinations that would provide information that might assist in decisions regarding risk and management.
   3. Orders necessary tests and medications essential to the conduct of anesthesia.
   4. Obtains consultations as necessary.
   5. Records impressions on the patient's chart.

C. Perianesthetic care means:
   1. Re-evaluation of patient immediately prior to induction.
   2. Preparation and check of equipment, drugs, fluids and gas supplies.
   3. Appropriate monitoring of the patient.
   4. Selection and administration of anesthetic agents to render the patient insensible to pain during the procedure.
   5. Support of life functions under the stress of anesthetic, surgical and obstetrical manipulations.
   6. Recording the event of the procedure.

Postanesthetic care means:
   1. The individual responsible for administering anesthesia remains with the patient as long as necessary.
   2. Availability of adequate nursing personnel and equipment necessary for safe postanesthetic are.
   3. Informing personnel caring for patients in the immediate postanesthetic period of any specific problems presented by each patient.
   4. Assurance that the patient is discharged in accordance with policies established by the Department of Anesthesiology.
   5. The period of postanesthetic surveillance is determined by the status of the patient and the judgment of the anesthesiologist. (Ordinarily, when a patient remains in the hospital postoperatively for 48 hours or longer, one or more notes should appear in addition to the discharge note from the postanesthesia care unit.)

Additional Areas of Expertise:

A. Resuscitation procedures.
B. Pulmonary care.
C. Critical (intensive) care.
D. Diagnosis and management of pain.
E. Trauma and emergency care.

Quality Assurance:

The anesthesiologist should participate in a planned program for evaluation of quality and appropriateness of patient care and resolving identified problems.

DOCUMENTATION OF ANESTHESIA CARE

(Approved by House of Delegates on October 12, 1988)

Documentation is a factor in the provision of quality care, and is the responsibility of an anesthesiologist. While anesthesia care is a continuum, it is usually viewed as consisting of preanesthesia, perianesthesia, and postanesthesia components. Anesthesia care should be documented to reflect these components and to facilitate review.

The record should include documentation of:

I. Preanesthesia Evaluation*

   A. Patient interview to review:
      1. Medical history
      2. Anesthesia history
      3. Medication history

   B. Appropriate Physical Examination.

   C. Review of objective diagnostic data (e.g. laboratory, ECG, X-ray).

   D. Assignment of ASA physical status.

   E. Formulation and discussion of an anesthesia plan with the patient and/ or responsible adult.

II. Perianesthesia (time-based record of events)

   A. Immediate review prior to initiation of anesthetic procedures:
      1. Patient re-evaluation
      2. Check of equipment, drugs and gas supply

   B. Monitoring of the patient** (e.g. recording of vital signs).

   C. Amounts of all drugs and agents used, and times given.

   D. The type and amounts of all intravenous fluids used including blood and blood products, and times given.

   E. The technique(s) used.

   F. Unusual events during the anesthesia period.

   G. The status of the patient at the conclusion of anesthesia.

III. Postanesthesia

A. Patient evaluation on admission and discharge from the post-anesthesia care unit.

B. A time-based record of vital signs and level of consciousness.

C. All drugs administered and their dosages.

D. Type and amounts of intravenous fluids administered including blood and blood products.

E. Any unusual events including post-anesthesia or post-procedural complications.

F. Post-anesthesia visits.

*See "Basic Standards for Preanesthesia Care"
**See "Standards for Basic Anesthetic Monitoring"

Reprinted with permission from reference 105.

Miscellaneous

Other Information

Example of Airway Assessment Procedures for Sedation and Analgesia

Positive pressure ventilation, with or without endotracheal intubation, may be necessary if respiratory compromise develops during sedation/ analgesia. This may be more difficult in patients with atypical airway anatomy. Also, some airway abnormalities may increase the likelihood of airway obstruction during spontaneous ventilation. Factors that may be associated with difficulty in airway management are:

History

- Previous problems with anesthesia or sedation
- Stridor, snoring, or sleep apnea
- Dysmorphic facial features (e.g., Pierre-Robin syndrome, trisomy 21)
- Advanced rheumatoid arthritis

Physical examination

- Habitus
  - Significant obesity (especially involving the neck and facial structures)
- Head and neck
  - Short neck, limited neck extension, decreased hyoid-mental distance (<3 cm in an adult), neck mass, cervical spine disease or trauma, tracheal deviation
- Mouth
  - Small opening (<3 cm in an adult); edentulous; protruding incisors; loose or capped teeth; high arched palate; macroglossia; tonsillar hypertrophy; nonvisible uvula
- Jaw
  - Micrognathia, retrognathia, trismus, significant malocclusion

Reprinted with permission from reference 106.

Example of Fasting Protocol for Sedation and Analgesia for Elective Procedures

Gastric emptying may be influenced by many factors, including anxiety, pain, abnormal autonomic function (e.g., diabetes), pregnancy, and mechanical obstruction. Therefore, the suggestions listed do not guarantee that complete gastric emptying has occurred. Unless contraindicated, pediatric patients should be offered clear liquids until 2-3 h before sedation to minimize the risk of dehydration.

	Solids and Nonclear Liquids*	Clear Liquids
Adults	6 - 8 h or none after midnight#	2 - 3 h
Children older than 36 months	6 - 8 h	2 - 3 h
Children aged 6-36 months	6 h	2 - 3 h
Children younger than 6 months	4 - 6 h	2 h

*This includes milk, formula, and breast milk (high fat content may delay gastric emptying).

#There are no data to establish whether a 6 - 8 h fast is equivalent to an overnight fast before sedation/analgesia.

Reprinted with permission from reference 106.

Example of Emergency Equipment for Sedation and Analgesia

Appropriate emergency equipment should be available whenever sedative or analgesic drugs capable of causing cardiorespiratory depression are administered. The table below should be used as a guide, which should be modified depending on the individual practice circumstances. Items in brackets are recommended when infants or children are sedated.

Intravenous equipment
- Gloves
- Tourniquets
- Alcohol wipes
- Sterile gauze pads
- Intravenous catheters [24- or 22-G]
- Intravenous tubing [pediatric "microdrip" (60 drops/ml)]
- Intravenous fluid
- Three-way stopcocks
- Assorted needles for drug aspiration, intramuscular injection [intraosseous bone marrow needle]
- Appropriately sized syringes
- Tape

Basic airway management equipment
- Source of compressed oxygen (tank with regulator or pipeline supply with flowmeter)
- Source of suction
- Suction catheters [pediatric suction catheters]
- Yankauer-type suction
- Face masks [infant/child]
- Self-inflating breathing bag-valve set [pediatric]
- Oral and nasal airways [infant/child-sized airways]
- Lubricant

Advanced airway management equipment (for practitioners with intubation skills)
- Laryngoscope handles (tested)
- Laryngoscope blades [pediatric]
- Endotracheal tubes
- Cuffed; 6.0, 7.0, or 8.0 mm ID [Uncuffed; 2.5, 3.0, 3.5, 4.0, 4.5, 5.0, 5.5, or 6.0 mm ID]
- Stylet (appropriately sized for endotracheal tubes)

Pharmacologic antagonists
- Naloxone
- Flumazenil

Emergency medications
- Epinephrine
- Ephedrine
- Atropine
- Lidocaine
- Glucose, 50% [10% or 25%]
- Diphenhydramine
- Hydrocortisone, methylprednisolone, or dexamethasone
- Diazepam or midazolam
- Ammonia spirits

Reprinted with permission from reference 106.

Example of Recovery and Discharge Criteria after Sedation and Analgesia

Each patient-care facility in which sedation/analgesia is administered should develop recovery and discharge criteria that are suitable for its specific patients and procedures. Some of the basic principles that might be incorporated in these criteria are enumerated.

General principles

1. All patients receiving sedation/analgesia should be monitored until appropriate discharge criteria are satisfied. The duration of monitoring must be individualized depending on the level of sedation achieved, overall condition of the patient, and nature of the intervention for which sedation/analgesia was administered.
2. The recovery area should be equipped with appropriate monitoring and resuscitation equipment.
3. A nurse or other trained individual should be in attendance until discharge criteria are fulfilled. An individual capable of establishing a patent airway and providing positive pressure ventilation should be immediately available.
4. Level of consciousness and vital signs (including frequency and depth of respiration in the absence of stimulation) should be recorded at regular intervals during recovery. The responsible practitioner should be notified if vital signs fall outside of the limits previously established for each patient.

Guidelines for discharge

1. Patients should be alert and oriented; infants and patients whose mental status was initially abnormal should have returned to their baseline. Practitioners must be aware that pediatric patients are at risk for airway obstruction should the head fall forward while the child is secured in a car seat.
2. Vital signs should be stable and within acceptable limits.
3. Sufficient Time (up to 2 h) should have elapsed after the last administration of reversal agents (naloxone, flumazenil) to ensure that patients do not become resedated after reversal effects have abated.
4. Outpatients should be discharged in the presence of a responsible adult who will accompany them home and be able to report any post-procedure complications.
5. Outpatients should be provided with written instructions regarding post-procedure diet, medications, and activities and a phone number to use in case of emergency.

Reprinted with permission from reference 106.

ACLS Protocols

Universal Algorithm for Adult Emergency Cardiac Care

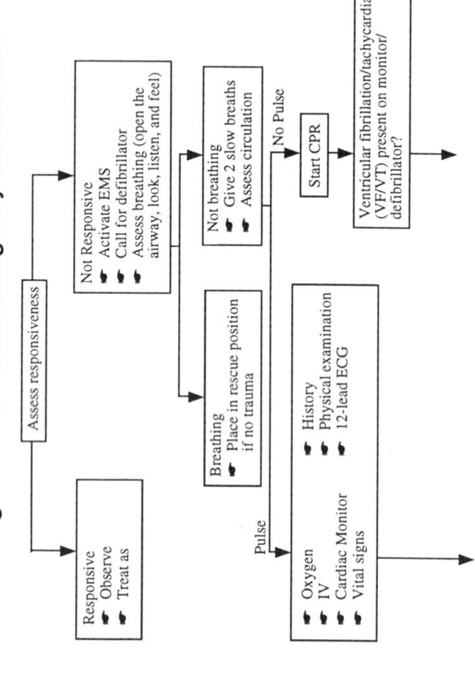

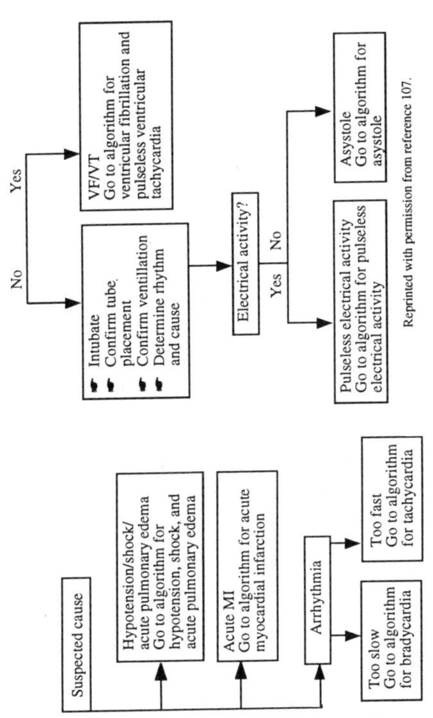

Reprinted with permission from reference 107.

Algorithm for Ventricular Fibrillation and Pulseless Ventricular Tachycardia

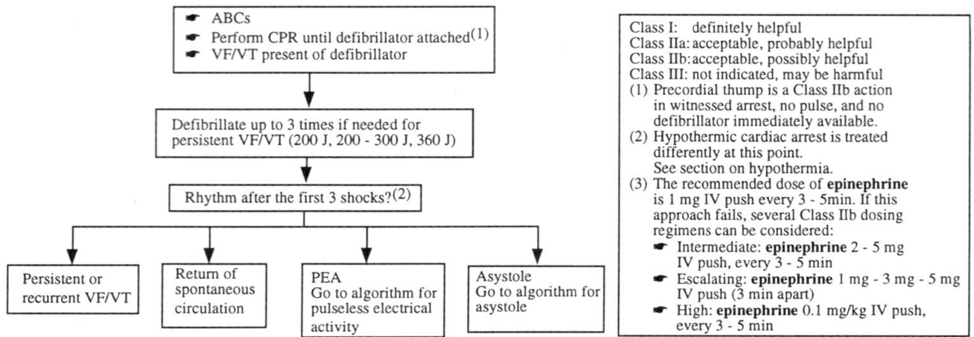

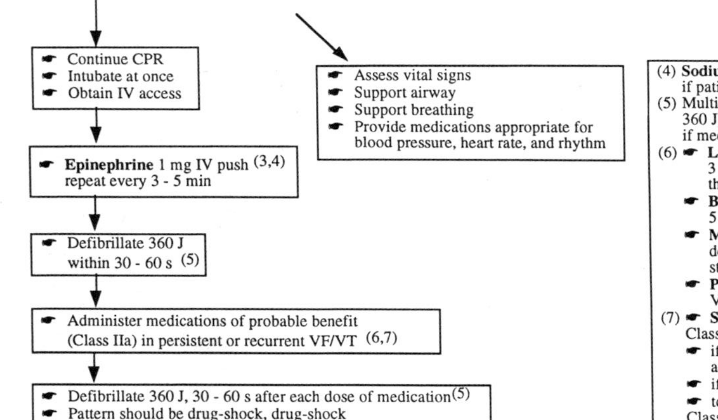

(4) **Sodium bicarbonate** (1 mEq/kg) is Class I if patient has known preexisting hyperkalemia

(5) Multiple sequenced shocks (200 J, 200 - 300 J, 360 J) are acceptable here (Class I), especially if medications are delayed

(6)
- **Lidocaine** 1.5 mg/kg IV push. Repeat in 3 - 5 min to total loading dose of 3 mg/kg; then use
- **Bretylium** 5 mg/kg IV push. Repeat in 5 min at 10 mg/kg
- **Magnesium sulfate** 1 - 2 g IV in torsades de pointes or suspected hypomagnesemic state or severe refractory VF
- **Procainamide** 30 mg/kg in refractory VF (maximum total 17 mg/kg)

(7)
- **Sodium bicarbonate** (1 mEq/kg IV):

Class IIa
- if known preexisting bicarbonate-sensitive acidosis
- if overdose of tricyclic antidepressants
- to alkalanize the urine in drug overdose

Class IIb
- if intubated and continued long arrest interval
- upon return of spontaneous circulation after long arrest interval

Class III
- hypoxic lactic acidosis

Reprinted with permission from reference 107.

Pulseless Electrial Activity (PEA) Algorithm

(Electromechanical Dissociation [EMD])

Includes

- Electromechanical dissociation (EMD)
- Pseudo-EMD
- Idioventricular rhythms
- Ventricular escape rhythms
- Bradyasystolic rhythms
- Postdefibrillation idioventricular rhythms

- Continue CPR
- Intubate at once
- Obtain IV access
- Assess blood flow using Doppler ultrasound, end-tidal CO_2, echocardiography, or arterial line

↓

Consider possible causes

(Parentheses = possible therapies and threatments)

- Hypovolemia (volume infusion)
- Hypoxia (ventilation)
- Cardiac tam-ponade (pericardiocentesis)
- Tension pneumothorax (needle decompression)
- Hypothermia (see hypothermia algorithm)
- Massive pulmonary embolism (surgery, **thrombolytics**)
- Drug overdoses such as tricyclics, digitalis, β-blockers, calcium channel blockers
- Hyperkalemia (1)
- Acidosis (2)
- Massive acute myocardial infarction (go to algorithm for massive acute MI)

↓

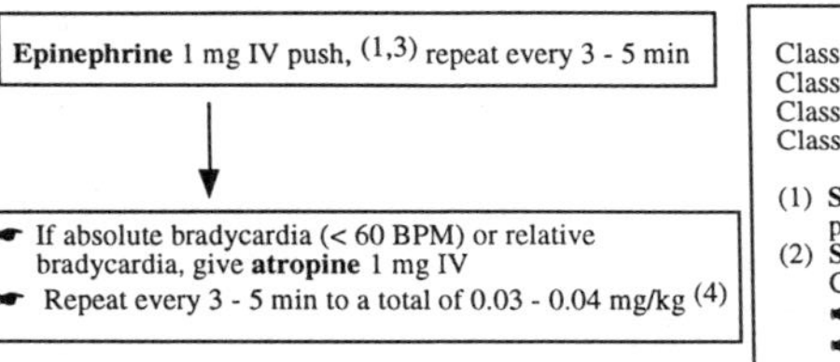

Class I: definitely helpful
Class IIa: acceptable, probably helpful
Class IIb: acceptable, possibly helpful
Class III: not indicated, may be harmful

(1) **Sodium bicarbonate** 1 mEq/ky is Class I if patient has known preexisting hyperkalemia.
(2) **Sodium bicarbonate** 1 mEq/kg:
  Class IIa
  - If known preexisting bicarbonate-responsive acidosis
  - If overdose with tricyclic antidepressants
  - To alkalinize urine in drug overdoses

  Class IIb
  - If intubated and continued long arrest interval
  - Upon return of spontaneous circulation after long arrest interval

  Class III
  - Hypoxic lactic acidosis

(3) The recommended dose is **epinephrine** is 1 mg IV push every 3 - 5 min. If this approach fails, several Class IIb dosing regimens can be considered:
  - Immediate: **epinephrine** 2 - 5 mg IV push, every 3 - 5 min
  - Escalating: **epinephrine** 1 mg - 3 mg - 5 mg IV push, 3 min apart
  - High: **epinephrine** 0.1 mg/kg IV push, every 3 - 5 min

(4) Shorter **atropine** dosing intervals (3 min) are possibly helpful in cardiac arrest (Class IIb).

Reprinted with permission from reference 107.

Asystole Treatment Algorithm

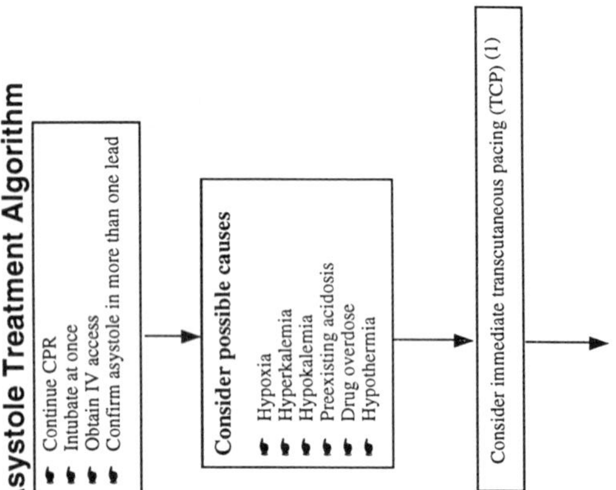

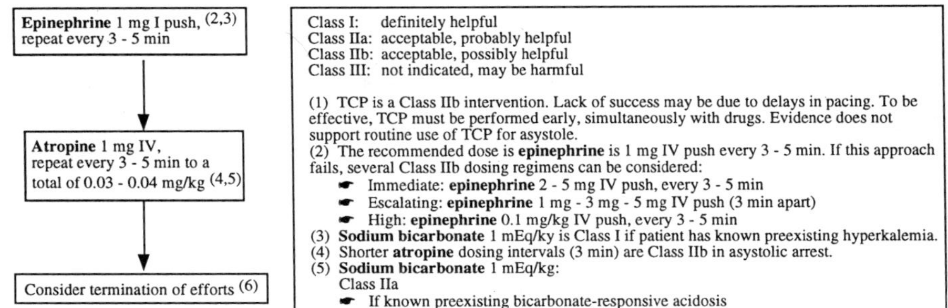

Reprinted with permission from reference 107.

Class I: definitely helpful
Class IIa: acceptable, probably helpful
Class IIb: acceptable, possibly helpful
Class III: not indicated, may be harmful

(1) TCP is a Class IIb intervention. Lack of success may be due to delays in pacing. To be effective, TCP must be performed early, simultaneously with drugs. Evidence does not support routine use of TCP for asystole.
(2) The recommended dose is **epinephrine** is 1 mg IV push every 3 - 5 min. If this approach fails, several Class IIb dosing regimens can be considered:
- Immediate: **epinephrine** 2 - 5 mg IV push, every 3 - 5 min
- Escalating: **epinephrine** 1 mg - 3 mg - 5 mg IV push (3 min apart)
- High: **epinephrine** 0.1 mg/kg IV push, every 3 - 5 min

(3) **Sodium bicarbonate** 1 mEq/ky is Class I if patient has known preexisting hyperkalemia.
(4) Shorter **atropine** dosing intervals (3 min) are Class IIb in asystolic arrest.
(5) **Sodium bicarbonate** 1 mEq/kg:
Class IIa
- If known preexisting bicarbonate-responsive acidosis
- If overdose with tricyclic antidepressants
- To alkalinize urine in drug overdoses

Class IIb
- If intubated and continued long arrest interval
- Upon return of spontaneous circulation after long arrest interval

Class III
- Hypoxic lactic acidosis

(6) If patient remains in asystole or other agonal rhythm after successful intubation and initial medications and no reversible causes are identified, consider termination of resuscitative efforts by a physician. Consider interval since arrest.

Bradycardia Algorithm

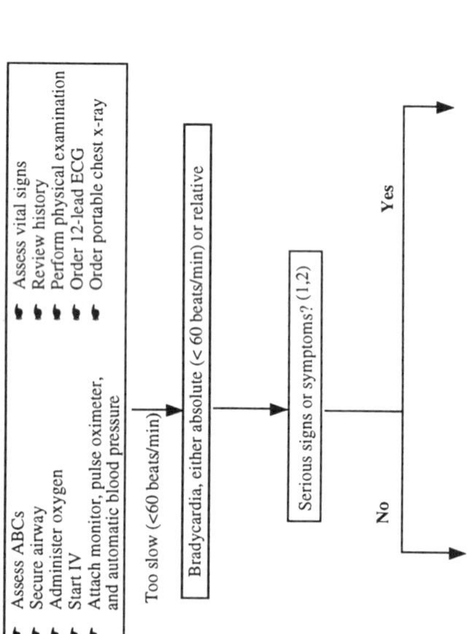

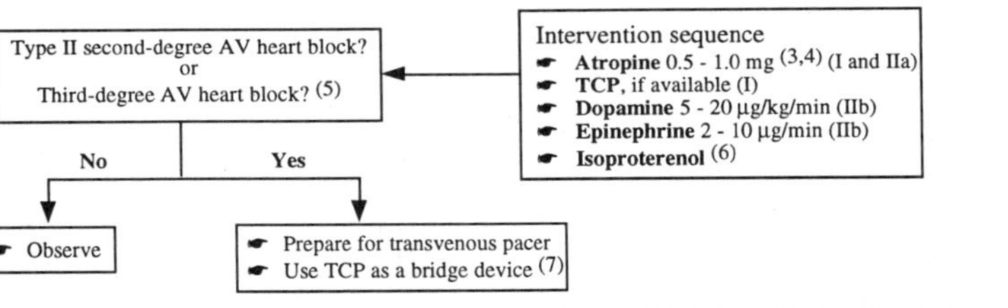

(1) Serious signs or symptoms must be related to the slow rate. Clinical manifestations include
- *Symptoms* (chest pain, shortness of breath, decrease level of consciousness) and
- *Signs* (low BP, shock, pulmonary congestion, CHF, acute MI)

(2) Do not delay TCP while awaiting IV access or for **atropine** to take effect if patient is symptomatic.

(3) Denervated transplanted hearts will not respond to **atropine**. Go at once to pacing, **catecholamine** infusion, or both.

(4) **Atropine** should be given in repeat doses every 3 - 5 min up to total of 0.03 - 0.04 mg/kg. Consider shorter dosing intervals (3 min) in severe clinical conditions. It has been suggested that **atropine** should be used with caution in atrioventricular (AV) block at the His-Purkinje level (type II AV block and new thrid-degree block with wide QRS complexes) (Class IIb).

(5). Never treat third-degree heart block plus ventricular escape beats with **lidocaine**.

(6) **Isoproterenol** should be used, if at all, with extreme caution. At low doses it is Class IIb (possibly helpful); at higher doses is is Class III (harmful).

(7) Verify patient tolerance and mechanical capture. Use analgesia and sedation as needed.

Reprinted with permission from reference 107.

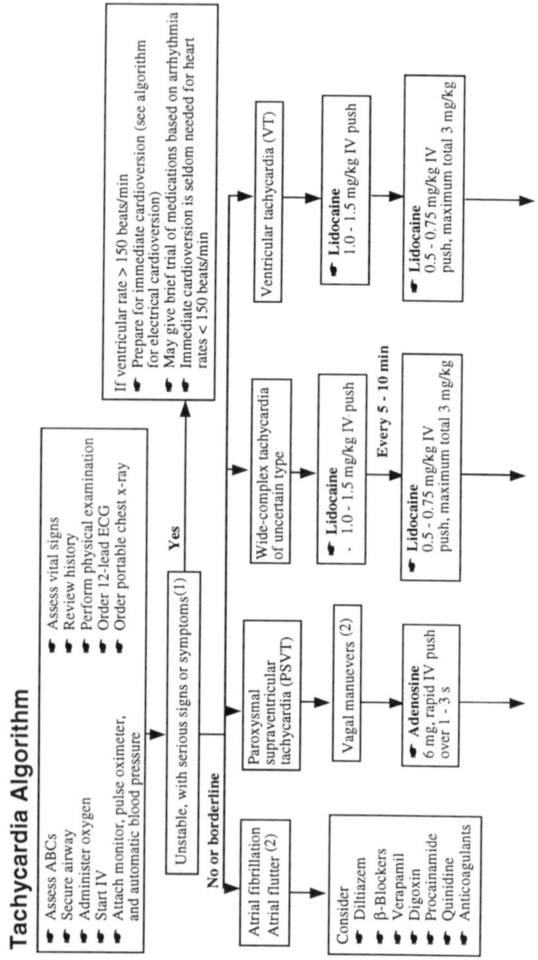

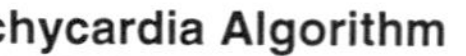

Tachycardia Algorithm

- Assess ABCs
- Secure airway
- Administer oxygen
- Start IV
- Attach monitor, pulse oximeter, and automatic blood pressure
- Assess vital signs
- Review history
- Perform physical examination
- Order 12-lead ECG
- Order portable chest x-ray

↓

Unstable, with serious signs or symptoms(1)

Yes →

If ventricular rate > 150 beats/min
- Prepare for immediate cardioversion (see algorithm for electrical cardioversion)
- May give brief trial of medications based on arrhythmia
- Immediate cardioversion is seldom needed for heart rates < 150 beats/min

No or borderline ↓

Atrial fibrillation
Atrial flutter (2)

↓

Consider
- Diltiazem
- β-Blockers
- Verapamil
- Digoxin
- Procainamide
- Quinidine
- Anticoagulants

Paroxysmal supraventricular tachycardia (PSVT)

↓

Vagal manuevers (2)

↓

- **Adenosine**
  6 mg, rapid IV push over 1 - 3 s

↓

Wide-complex tachycardia of uncertain type

↓

- **Lidocaine**
  1.0 - 1.5 mg/kg IV push

↓ **Every 5 - 10 min**

- **Lidocaine**
  0.5 - 0.75 mg/kg IV push, maximum total 3 mg/kg

↓

Ventricular tachycardia (VT)

↓

- **Lidocaine**
  1.0 - 1.5 mg/kg IV push

↓

- **Lidocaine**
  0.5 - 0.75 mg/kg IV push, maximum total 3 mg/kg

↓

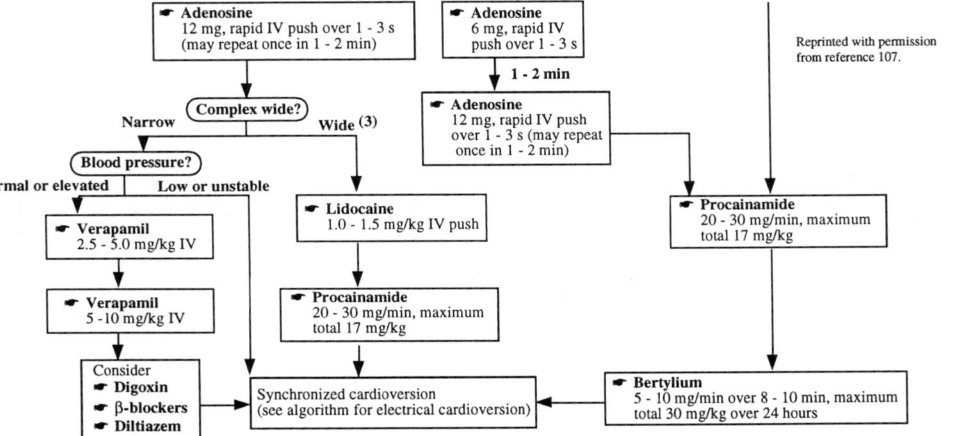
Adenosine
12 mg, rapid IV push over 1 - 3 s
(may repeat once in 1 - 2 min)
Adenosine
6 mg, rapid IV
push over 1 - 3 s
1 - 2 min
Adenosine
12 mg, rapid IV push
over 1 - 3 s (may repeat
once in 1 - 2 min)
Reprinted with permission
from reference 107.
Complex wide?
Narrow
Wide (3)
Blood pressure?
Normal or elevated
Low or unstable
Verapamil
2.5 - 5.0 mg/kg IV
Verapamil
5 -10 mg/kg IV
Consider
Digoxin
β-blockers
Diltiazem
Lidocaine
1.0 - 1.5 mg/kg IV push
Procainamide
20 - 30 mg/min, maximum
total 17 mg/kg
Procainamide
20 - 30 mg/min, maximum
total 17 mg/kg
Synchronized cardioversion
(see algorithm for electrical cardioversion)
Bertylium
5 - 10 mg/min over 8 - 10 min, maximum
total 30 mg/kg over 24 hours
(1) Ustable condition must be related to tachycardia. Signs and symptoms may include chest pain, shortness of breath, decreaed level of consciousness, low blood pressure (BP), shock, pulmonary congestion, congestive heart failure, acute myocardial infarction.
(2) Carotid sinus pressure is contraindicated in patients with carotid bruits; avoid ice water immersion in patients with ischemic heart disease.
(3) If the wide-complex tachycardia is known with certainty to be PSVT and BP is normal/elevated, sequence can include verapamil.
(4) Use extreme caution with β-blockers after verapamil.

Electrical Cardioversion Algorithm
(with the patient is not in cardiac arrest)

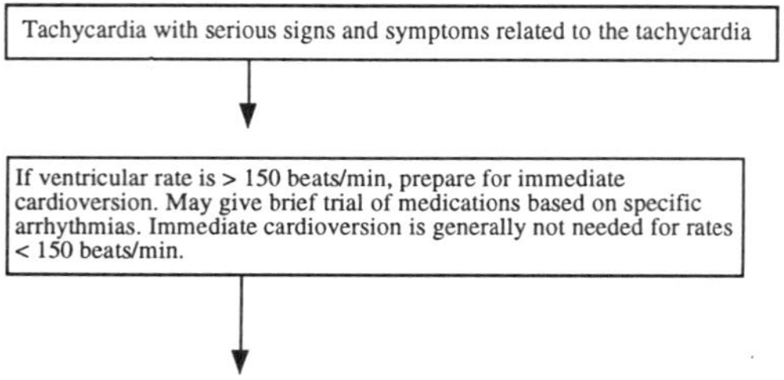

Tachycardia with serious signs and symptoms related to the tachycardia

↓

If ventricular rate is > 150 beats/min, prepare for immediate cardioversion. May give brief trial of medications based on specific arrhythmias. Immediate cardioversion is generally not needed for rates < 150 beats/min.

↓

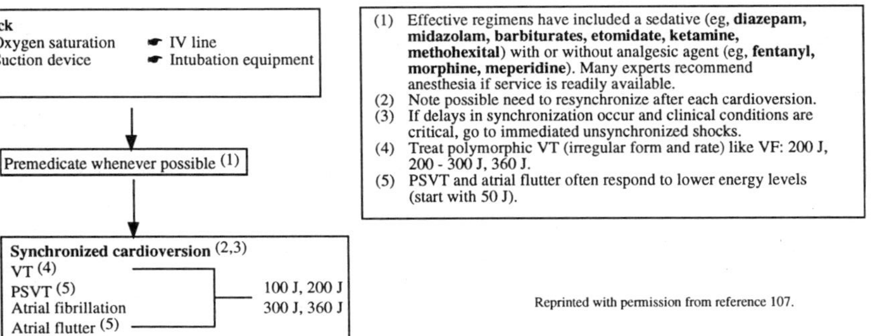

Reprinted with permission from reference 107.

Algorithm for Hypotension, Shock, and Acute Pulmonary Edema

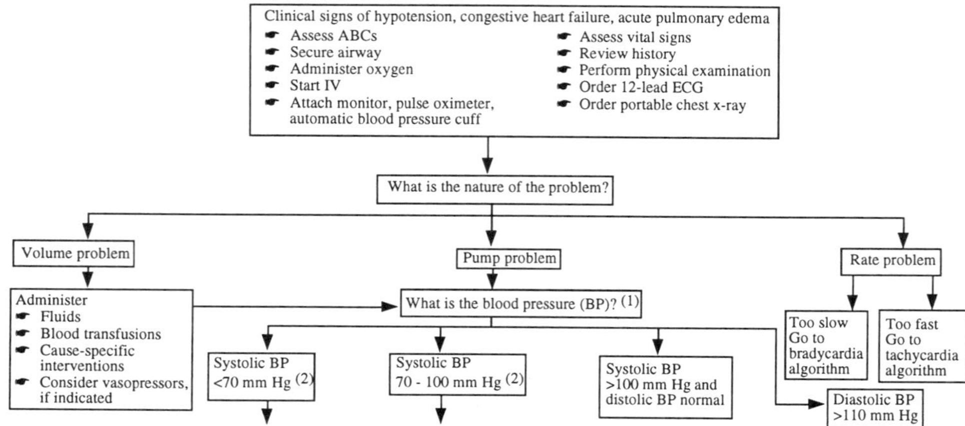

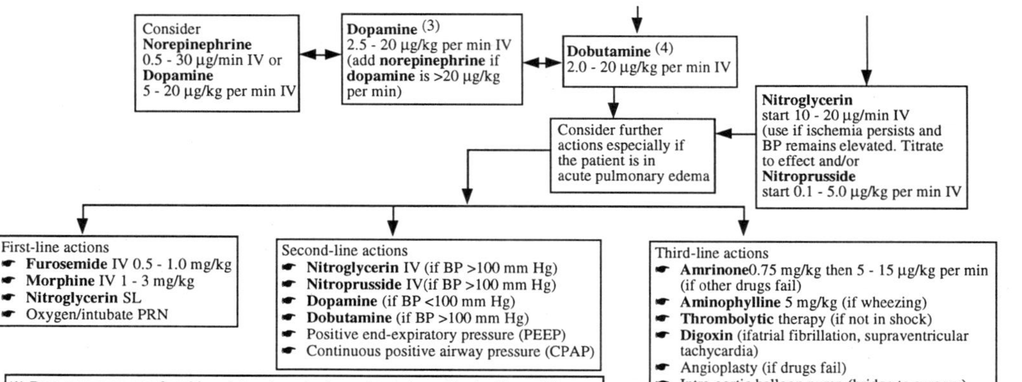

Reprinted with permission from reference 107.

Acute Myocardial Infarction (AMI) Algorithm

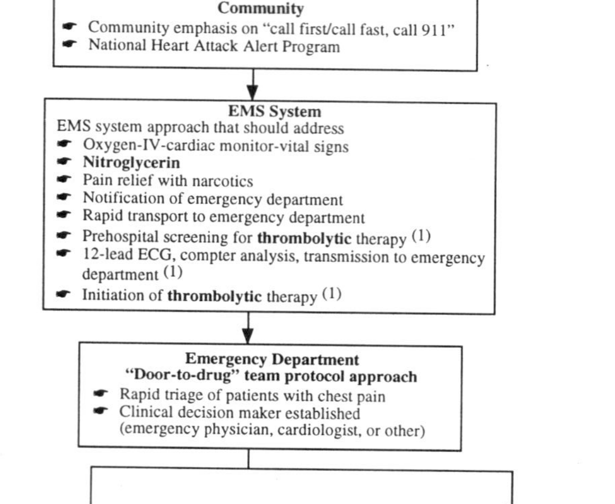

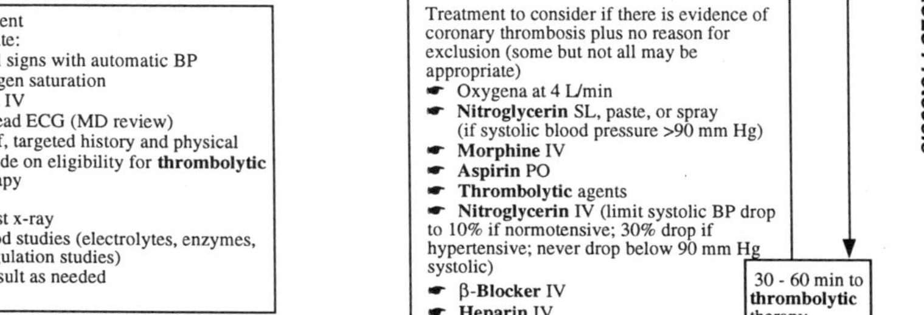

Reprinted with permission from reference 107.

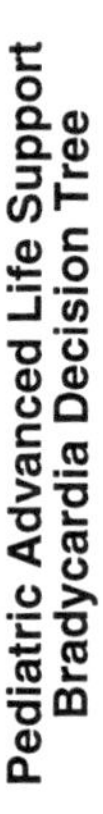
Pediatric Advanced Life Support
Bradycardia Decision Tree

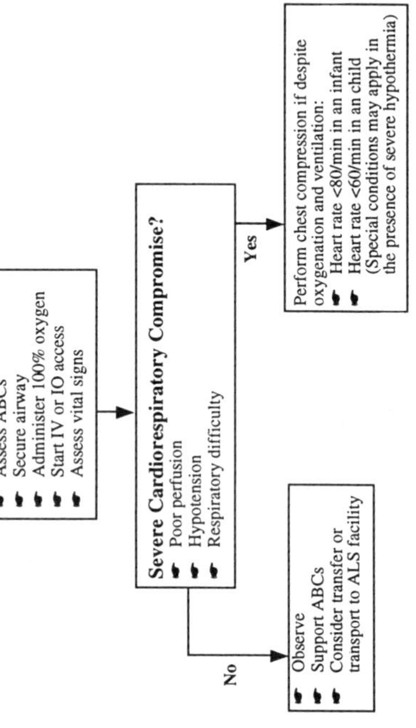
Assess ABCs
Secure airway
Administer 100% oxygen
Start IV or IO access
Assess vital signs
Severe Cardiorespiratory Compromise?
Poor perfusion
Hypotension
Respiratory difficulty
No
Observe
Support ABCs
Consider transfer or transport to ALS facility
Yes
Perform chest compression if despite oxygenation and ventilation:
Heart rate <80/min in an infant
Heart rate <60/min in an child
(Special conditions may apply in the presence of severe hypothermia)

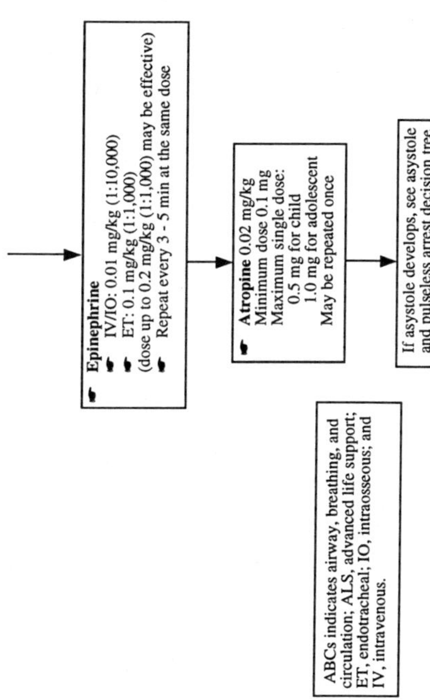

Reprinted with permission from reference 108.

Pediatric Advanced Life Support
Asystole and Pulseless Arrest Decision Tree

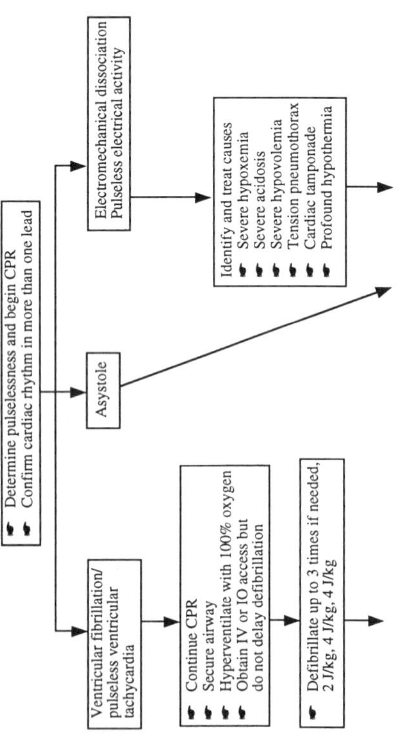

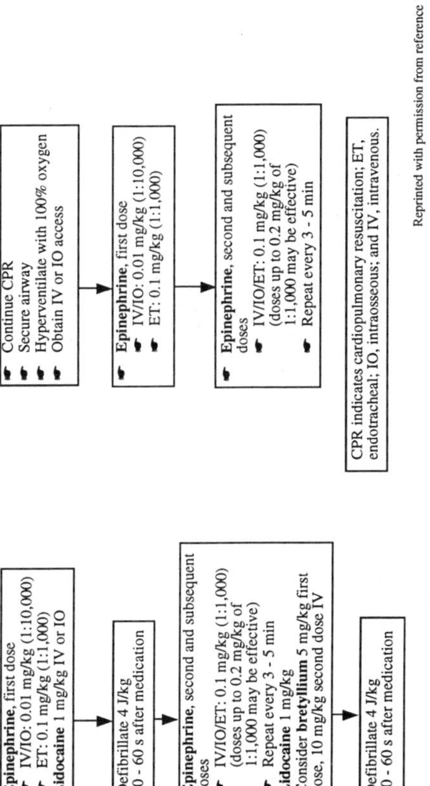

Reprinted with permission from reference 108.

1 Courtesy of Dr. W. T. Ross, Department of Anesthesiology, University of Virginia Medical School, Charlottesville, Virginia

2 Zaidan JR. Electrocardiography. In Clinical Anesthesia (2nd edition, Barash PG, Cullen BF, Stoelting RK, eds.) Philadelphia, JB Lippincott, 1992; 771-805

3 London MJ, Hollenberg M, Wong, et al. Intraoperative Myocardial Ischemia: Localization by Continuous 12-Lead Electrocardiography. Anesthesiology 1988; 69:232-41

4 Goldman L, Caldera DL, Nussbaum SR, et al. Multifactorial Index of Cardiac Risk in Noncardiac Surgical Procedures. N Engl J Med 1977; 297:845-50.

5 Eagle KA, Brundage BH, Chaitma BR, et al. Guidelines for Perioperative Cardiovascular Evaluation for Noncardiac Surgery. Circulation 1996; 93:1278-317

6 Mangano ST, Goldman L. Preoperative Assessment of Patients with Known or Suspected Coronary Disease. N Engl J Med 1995; 333:1750-6

7 Atlee JL. Arrhythmias and Pacemakers. Practical Management for Anesthesia and Critical Care Medicine. Philadelphia, WB Saunders, 1996

8 Anonymous. Prevention of Wound Infection and Sepsis in Surgical Patients. Medical Letter 1993; 35:91-4

9 Dajani AS, Bisno AL, Chung KJ, et al. Prevention of Bacterial Endocarditis; Recommendations by the American Heart Association. JAMA 1990; 264: 2919-22

10 Anonymous. FDA Anesthesia Apparatus Checkout Recommendations. Anesthesia Patient Safety Foundation Newsletter, 1994; 9:36

11 Ehrenwerth J, Eisenkraft JB. Anesthesia Equipment: Principles and Applications. St. Louis, Mosby-Year Book; 1993

12 Dorsch JA, Dorsch SE. Understanding Anesthesia Equipment: Construction, Care and Complications (2nd ed.) Baltimore, Williams and Wilkins, 1984

13 Conway CM. Anaesthetic Breathing Systems. Br J Anaesth 1985; 57:649-57

14 Anonymous. Report of the Second Task Force on Blood Pressue Control in Children - 1987. Task Force on Blood Pressure Control in Children. Pediatrics 1987; 79:1-27

15 Atlee JL. Perioperative Cardiac Dysrhythmias: Mechanisms, Recognition, Management. Chicago, Year Book Medical Publishers, 1985

16 Meakin G. Neonatal Anesthetic Pharmacology. In Handbook of Neonatal Anaesthesia (Hughes D, Mather S, Wolf A., eds.). London, WB Saunders, 1996;18-54

17 Bruce DL, Linde HW. Vaporization of Mixed Anesthetic Liquids. Anesthesiology 1984; 60:342-6

18 Noren RL. Opiate Pharmacology. In Handbook of Critical Care Pain Management (Hamill RJ, Rowlingson JC, eds.) New York, McGraw-Hill, 1994;117-41

19 Ramadhyani U. Opioids and Nonopioid Analgesics. In Practical Anesthetic Pharmacology (2nd edition, Attia RR, Grogono AW, Domer FR, eds) Norwalk, Connecticut, Appleton-Century-Crofts, 1987;107-32

20 Kahana M. Pain Management in the Critically Ill Child. In Handbook of Critical Care Pain Management (Hamill RJ, Rowlingson JC, eds.) New York, McGraw-Hill, 1994;507-21

21 Benedetti C, Butler SH. Systemic analgesics. In The Management of Pain (2nd ed,Bonica JJ, ed.), Philadelphia, Lea & Febiger, 1990;1640-75

22 Lee VC, Rowlingson JC, Hammil RJ. Nonsteroidal Analgesic and Anti-inflammatory Agents. In Handbook of Critical Care Pain Management (Hamill RJ, Rowlingson JC, eds.) New York, McGraw-Hill, 1994;103-15

23 Attia RR, Gorgono AW, Domer FR. Psychotropic Agents In Practical Anesthetic Pharmacology (2nd edition, Attia RR, Grogono AW, Domer FR, eds) Norwalk, Connecticut, Appleton-Century-Crofts, 1987;149-69

24 Attia RR, Gorgono AW, Domer FR. Sedative-Hypnotics and Antiepileptics In Practical Anesthetic Pharmacology (2nd edition, Attia RR, Grogono AW, Domer FR, eds) Norwalk, Connecticut, Appleton-Century-Crofts, 1987;133-48

25 Yaster M, Maxwell LG. Pediatric Regional Anesthesia. Anesthesiology 1989; 70:324-38

26 Youngberg JA. Intravenous Induction Agents In Practical Anesthetic Pharmacology (2nd edition, Attia RR, Grogono AW, Domer FR, eds) Norwalk, Connecticut, Appleton-Century-Crofts, 1987;39-53

27 Attia RR, Gorgono AW, Domer FR. Drugs that Affect the Autonomic Nervous SystemIn Practical Anesthetic Pharmacology (2nd edition, Attia RR, Grogono AW, Domer FR, eds) Norwalk, Connecticut, Appleton-Century-Crofts, 1987;171-93

28 Graf G, Rosenbaum S. Anesthesia and the Endocrine System. In Clinical Anesthesia (2nd edition, Barash PG, Cullen BF, Stoelting RK, eds.) Philadelphia, JB Lippincott, 1992;1237-65.

29 Zimmer JL. Hypertensive Crises: Emergencies and Urgencies. In Textbook of Critical Care (3rd edition, Ayres SM, Grenvik A, Holbrook PR, Shoemaker WC, eds) Philadelphia, WB Saunders, 1995;522-38

30 Anonymous. Drugs of Choice for Common Arrhythmias. The Medical Letter 1996; 38:75-82

31 Bonica JJ, Buckley FP. Regional Analgesia with Local Anesthetics. In The Management of Pain (2nd edition; Bonica JJ, ed.) Philadelphia, Lea & Febiger, 1990;1883-966

32 DiFazio CA, Rowlingson JC. Regional Anesthesia and Postoperative Analgesia. In Anesthetic Management of Difficult and Routine Pediatric Patients (Berry FA, ed.) New York, Churchill Livingston, 1986;389-406

33 Davis WJ, Lennon RL. Outpatient Surgery. In Orthopedic Anesthesia (Wedel DJ, ed.) New York, Churchill Livingstone, 1993;233-54

34 Anonymous. Practice guidelines for management of the difficult airway. A report by the American Society of Anesthesiologists Task Force on Management of the Difficult Airway. Anesthesiology 1993; 78:597-602

35 Cormack RS, Lehane J. Difficult Tracheal Intubation in Obstetrics. Anaesthesia 1984; 39:1105-11

36 Mallampati SR, Gatt SP, Gugino LD, et al. A Clinical Sign to Predict Difficult Tracheal Intubation: A Prospective Study. Can J Anesth 1985; 32:429-34

37 Benumof JL. Airway Management Principles and Practice. St. Louis, Mosby-Year Book, 1995

38 Pontpoppidan H, Geffin B, Lowenstein E. Objective Quantitative Criteria for Tracheal Intubation. N Engl J Med 1972; 287:743-52

39 Benumof JL. Laryngeal Mask Airway and the ASA Difficult Airway Algorithm. Anesthesiology 1996; 84:686-99

40 Mihm FG, Rosenthal MH. Pulmonary Artery Catherization. In Clinical Procedures in Anesthesia and Intensive Care (Benumof JL, ed.) Philadelphia, JB Lippincott, 1992;405-42

41 Varon AJ. Hemodynamic Monitoring: Arterial and Pulmonary Artery Catheters. In Critical Care (2nd edition; Civetta JM, Taylor RW, Kirby, RR, eds.) Philadelphia, JB Lippincott, 1992;255-69

42 Daily EK, Schroeder JS (eds.): Techniques in Bedside Hemodynamic Monitoring, St. Louis, C.V. Mosby, 1985

43 Fugate JH, Todres ID. Central Venous Cannulation. In Critical Care of Infants and Children (Todres ID, Fugate JH, eds) Boston, Little, Brown, 1996;51-8

44 Moore RA, Martin DE. Anesthetic Management of Valvular Heart Disease. In The Practice of Cardiac Anesthesia (Hensley FA, Martin DE, eds.) Boston, Little, Brown, 1990:350-85

45 Lake C. Cardiovascular Diseases. In Pediatrics for the Anesthesiologist (Berry FA, Steward DJ, eds.) New York, Churchill Livingston, 1993;25-66

46 Weisberg LS, Szerlip HM, Cox M. Disorders of Potassium Homeostasis in Critically Ill Patients. In Critical Care Clinics (Geheb M, Carlson R, eds) Philadelphia, W.B. Saunders 1987; 3:835-54

47 Link D. Fluids, Electrolytes, Acid-Base Disturbances, and Diuretics. In Critical Care of Infants and Children (Todres ID, Fugate JH, eds) Boston, Little, Brown, 1996;410-35

48 Anonymous. Practice Guidelines for Pulmonary Artery Catheterization. A Report by the American Society of Anesthesiologists Task Force on Pulmonary Artery Catheterization. Anesthesiology 1993; 78:380-94

49 Anonymous. Practice Guidelines for Perioperative Transesophageal Echocardiography. A Report by the American Society of Anesthesiologists and the Society of Cardiovascular Anesthesiologists Task Force on Transesophageal Echocardiography. Anesthesiology 1996; 84:986-1006

50 Bendo AA, Hartung J, Kass IS, Cottrell JE. Neurophysiology and Neuroanesthesia. In Clinical Anesthesia (2nd edition, Barash PG, Cullen BF, Stoelting RK, eds.) Philadelphia, JB Lippincott, 1992;871-918

51 Pasterneck M. Infections of the Central Nervous System. In Critical Care of Infants and Children (Todres ID, Fugate JH, eds.) Boston, Little, Brown, 1996;385-95

52 Dooling EC. Coma. In Critical Care of Infants and Children (Todres ID, Fugate JH, eds.) Boston, Little, Brown, 1996;374-7

53 Harris M. Neurologic and Neuromuscular Diseases. In Pediatrics for the Anesthesiologist (Berry FA, Steward DJ, eds.) New York, Churchill Livingston, 1993;197-220

54 Prough DS. Brain Monitoring. In: Critical Care: State of the Art. (Shoemaker W, Taylor R, eds.) Fullerton, CA, Society of Critical Care Medicine, 1991; 12:158-70

55 Deyo DJ, Prough DS. Brain Function Monitoring. In Textbook of Critical Care (3rd edition, Ayres SM, Grenvik A, Holbrook PR, Shoemaker WC, eds) Philadelphia, WB Saunders, 1995:321-xxx

56 Scott GM, Steward DJ. Diseases of the Endocrine System. In Pediatrics for the Anesthesiologist (Berry FA, Steward DJ, eds.) New York, Churchill Livingston, 1993;155-96

57 Pickett JA, Wheeldon D, Odura A. Multi-organ Transplantation: Donor Management. Current Opinion in Anaesthesiology Philadelphia, Current Science 1994;7 :80-3

58 Anonymous. Questions and Answers about Transfusion Practices (2nd edition), American Society of Anesthesiologists Committee on Transfusion Medicine, 1992

59 Ritter DF, Sarsnic MA. Transfusion Therapy Part I. Progress in Anesthesiology 1989; 3:1-14

60 Sayers MH, McAuthur J, McDonald JS. The Hematology of Pregnancy. In Principles and Practice of Obstetric Analgesia and Anesthesia (2nd edition; Bonica JJ, McDonald JS, eds.) Baltimore, Williams & Wilkins, 1995;1096-119

61 Jandl JH. Blood Textbook of Hematology, Boston, Little, Brown, 1996

62 Erban SB, Kinman JL, Schwartz JS. Routine Use of the Prothrombin and Partial Thromboplastin Times. JAMA 1989; 262:2428-32

63 Mallett SV, Cox DJA. Thrombelastography. Br J Anaesth 1992; 69:307-13

64 Hirsh J, Hoak J. Management of Deep Vein Thrombosis and Pulmonary Embolism. Circulation 1996; 93:2212-45

65 JT Herrin. The Kidney. In JF Burke (ed.): Surgical Physiology. Philadelphia, WB Saunders, 1983;187-207

66 Levy JH. Anaphylactic Reactions in Anesthesia and Intensive care (2nd edition), Stoneham, MA, Butterworth and Heinemann, 1992

67 Astra USA, Inc., 50 Otis Street, Westborough, MA 01581-4500

68 Buroni P. Anatomy. In Regional Anesthesia in Children (Saint-Marice C, Steinberg OS, eds.) Fribourgl, Switzerland, Mediglobe, 1990;16-25

69 Peterfreund RA, Datta S. Ostheimer G: pH Adjustment of Local Anesthetic Solutions with Sodium Bicarbonate: Laboratory Evaluation of Alkalinization and Precipitation. Reg Anesth 1989; 14(2S):74

70 Bosenberg A. Difficult Intubation in Neonates and Small Infants. In Handbook of Neonatal Anaesthesia (Hughes D, Mather S, Wolf A., eds.) London, WB Saunders, 1996:298-330

71 Woods AM. Pediatric Endoscopy. In Anesthetic Management of Difficult and Routine Pediatric Patients (2nd edition; Berry FA, ed.) New York, Churchill Livingston, 1990:199-242

72 Berry FA. Acute Airway Obstruction, with Special Emphasis on Epiglottitis and Croup. In Anesthetic Management of Difficult and Routine Pediatric Patients (2nd edition; Berry FA, ed.) New York, Churchill Livingston, 1990:243-65.

73 Textbook of Neonatal Resuscitation. Dallas, American Heart Association, 1994

74 Berry FA. Practical Aspects of Fluid and Electrolyte Therapy. In Anesthetic Management of Difficult and Routine Pediatric Patients (2nd edition; Berry FA, ed.) New York, Churchill Livingston, 1990:89-120

75 Siegel NJ, Carpenter T, Gandio KM. The Pathophysiology of Body Fluids. In Principle and Practice of Pediatrics (2nd edition, Oski, FA, DeAngelis CD, Feigin RD, et al, eds.) Philadelphia, JB Lippincott, 1994;60-79

76 Jones AEP, Pelton DA. An Index of Syndromes and Their Anesthetic Implications. Can J Anesth 1976; 23:207-26

77 Check TG, Gutche, B. Maternal Physiologic Alterations during Pregnancy. In Anesthesia for Obstetrics (3rd edition; Shnider SM, Levinson, G., eds.) Baltimore, Williams and Wilkins; 1993:3-17

78 Bonica JJ. Maternal Anatomic and Physiologic Alterations During Pregnancy and Parturition. In Principles and Practice of Obstetric Analgesia and Anesthesia (McDonald JS, ed.) Baltimore, Williams & Wilkins; 1995:45-82

79 Conklin KA. Physiologic Changes of Pregnancy. In Obstetric Anesthesia Principles and Practice (Chestnut DH, ed.) St. Louis, Mosby; 1994:17-42

80 Pritchard JA, MacDonald PC, Gant NF. Williams Obstetrics (17th edition), Norwalk, Connecticut , Appleton-Century-Crofts, 1985

81 Clark SB, Cotton DB. Clinical Indications for Pulmonary Artery Catheterization in the Patient with Severe Preeclampsia. Am J. Obstet Gynecol 1988; 158:453-8

82 Pederson H, Santos AC, Finster M. Obstetric Anesthesia. In Clinical Anesthesia (2nd edition; Barash PG, Cullen BF, Stoelting RK, eds.) Philadelphia, JB Lippincott, 1992:1215-51

83 Gutsche BB, Cheek TG. Anesthetic Considerations in Preeclampsia-Eclampsia. In Anesthesia for Obstetrics (3rd edition; Shnider SM, Levinson G., eds.) Baltimore, Williams and Wilkins; 1993:305-36

84 Reisner LC, Lin D. Anesthesia for Cesarean Section. In Obstetric Anesthesia Principles and Practice (Chestnut DH, ed.) St. Louis, Mosby; 1994:459-86

85 Parer JT. Diagnosis and Management of Fetal Asphyxia. In Anesthesia for Obstetrics (3nd edition; Shnider SM, Levinson G, eds.) 1993:657-70

86 Friedman EA, Patterns of Labor as Indicators of Risk. Clin Obstet Gynecol 1973; 16:172-83

87 Zlatnik FJ. Normal labor and delivery and its conduct. In Danforth's Obstetrics and Gynecology (6th edition, Scott JR, DiSaia PJ, Hammond CB, Spellacy WN, eds.) Philadelphia, JB Lippincott 1994:105-28

88 Pernoll ML, Mandell JE. Cesarean Section. In Principles and Practice of Obstetric Analgesia and Anesthesia (McDonald JS, ed.), Baltimore, Williams & Wilkins, 1995, 968-1009

89 Harris AP. Emergency Cesarean Section. In Current Practice in Anesthesiology (Rogers MC, ed.) Toronto, BC Decker, 1990:361-6

90 Campbell C. Steps to Minimize Pulmonary Aspiration in the Obstetric Patient. In Challenges in Clinical Anesthesia Updates Philadelphia, Lippincott 1993;4:1-6

91 Shnider SM, Levinson G. Anesthesia for Cesarean Section. In Anesthesia for Obstetrics (3nd edition; Shnider SM, Levinson G, eds.) 1993:211-46

92 Conklin KA. PhysiologicChanges of Pregnancy. In Obstetric Anesthesia Principles and Practice (Chestnut, DH, ed.) St. Louis, MO, Mosby-Year Book, 1994, 17-42

93 Naulty JS. Epidural Analgesia for Labor. In Obstetric Anesthesia. (Norris, MC, ed.) Philadelphia, JB Lippincott 1993:319-40

94 Pedersen H, Santos AC, Finster M. Obstetric Anesthesia. In Clinical Anesthesia (2nd edition, Barash PG, Cullen BF, Stoelting RK, eds.) Philadelphia, JB Lippincott, 1992;1215-51

95 Anonymous. Practice Guidelines for Acute Pain Management in the Perioperative Setting. A Report by the American Society of Anesthesiologists Task Force on Pain Management, Acute Pain Section. Anesthesiology 1995; 82:1071-81

96 Edwards WT, Peeters-Asdourian C. Systemic Pharmacologic Approaches. In Principles and Practice of Pain Management (Warfield, CA, ed.) McGraw-Hill, New York, NY 1994:349-61

97 Anonymous. Practice Guidelines for Cancer Pain Management. A Report by the American Society of Anesthesiologists Task Force on Pain Management, Cancer Pain Section. Anesthesiology; 84:1243-57

98 Gracely GH, Price DD, Roberts WJ, Bennett GJ. Quantitative Sensory Testing in Patients with Complex Regional Pain Syndrome (CRPS) I and II. In Reflex Sympathetic Dystrophy: A Reappraisal (Jaenig W, Stanton-Hicks M, eds.) Seattle, IASP Press, 1996:151-72

99 Boas RA. Complex Regional Pain Syndromes: Symptoms, Signs, and Differential Diagnosis. In Reflex Sympathetic Dystrophy: A Reappraisal (Jaenig W, Stanton-Hicks M, eds.) Seattle, IASP Press, 1996:79-92

100 Baron R, Blumberg H, Jaenig W. Clinical Characteristics of Patients with Complex Regional Pain Syndrome in Germant with Special Emphasis on Vasomotor Function. In Reflex Sympathetic Dystrophy: A Reappraisal (Jaenig W, Stanton-Hicks M, eds.) Seattle, IASP Press, 1996:25-48

101 Wilder RT. Reflex Symphathetic Dystrophy in Children and Adolescents: Differences with Adults. In Reflex Sympathetic Dystrophy: A Reappraisal (Jaenig W, Stanton-Hicks M, eds.) Seattle, IASP Press, 1996:67-78

102 Wilson PR, Low PA, Bedder MD, Covington EC, Rauck RL. Diagnostic Algorithm for Complex Regional Pain Syndromes. In Reflex Sympathetic Dystrophy: A Reappraisal (Jaenig W, Stanton-Hicks M, eds.) Seattle, IASP Press, 1996:93-106.

103 Stanton-Hicks M, Raj PP, Racz GB. Use of Regional Anesthetics for Diagnosis of Reflex Sympathetic Dystrophy and Sympathetically Maintained Pain: A Critical Evaluation. In Reflex Sympathetic Dystrophy: A Reappraisal (Jaenig W, Stanton-Hicks M, eds.) Seattle, IASP Press, 1996:217-38

104 Malignant Hyperthermia Association of the United States (MHAUS), Westport, CT

105 Standards and Guidelines from "ASA Standards, Guidelines and Statements" (October, 1993). Reproduced with permission from the American Society of Anesthesiologist

106 Anonymous. Practice Guidelines for Sedation and Analgesia by Non-anesthesiologists. A Report by the American Society of Anesthesiologists Task Force on Sedation and Analgesia by Non-Anesthesiologists. Anesthesiology 1996; 84:459-71

107 Guidelines for Cardiopulmonary Resuscitation and Emergency Cardiac Care. Emergency Cardiac Care Committee and Subcommittees, American Heart Association. Part VII. Advanced Life Support. JAMA 1992; 268;2199-241

108 Guidelines for Cardiopulmonary Resuscitation and Emergency Cardiac Care. Emergency Cardiac Care Committee and Subcommittees, American Heart Association. Part VII. Pediatric Advanced Life Support. JAMA 1992; 268;2262-75